腎臟醫學
臨床技能手冊

The Handbook of Clinical Skills
in Nephrology, 2nd Edition

第二版

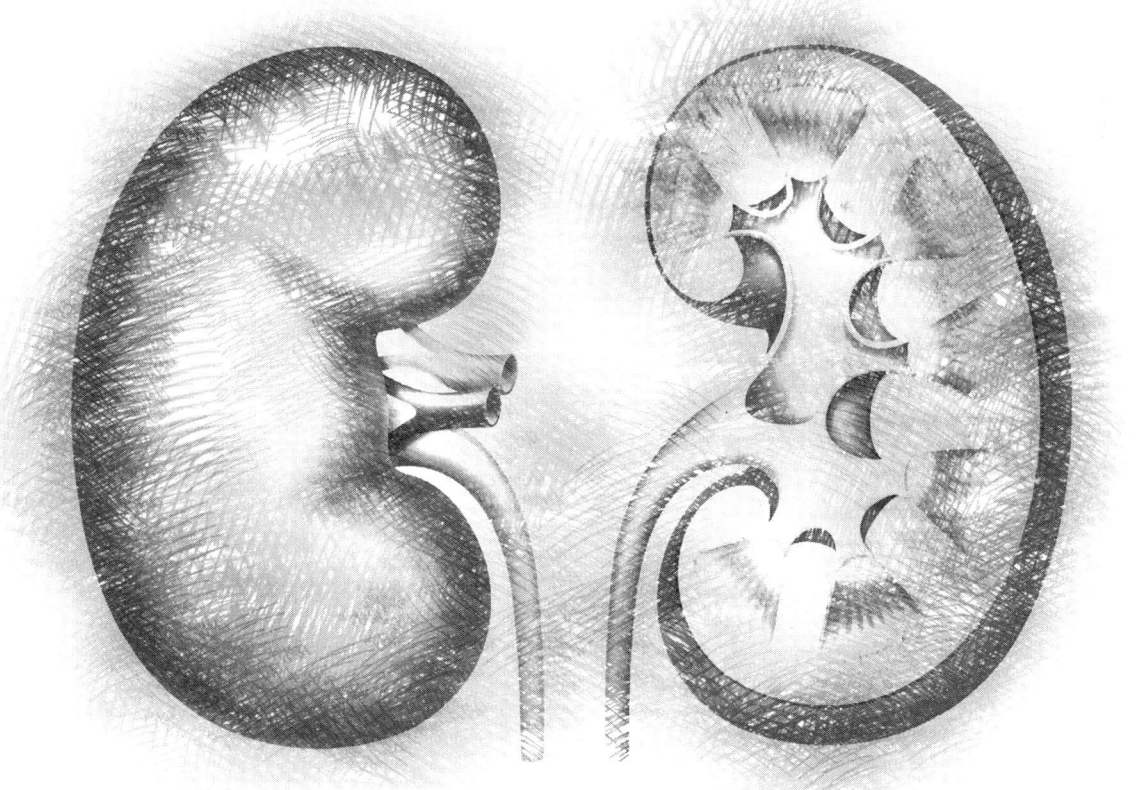

唐德成、林志慶 主編

序

臺北榮民總醫院是國家級醫學中心，除臨床服務與研究創新外，亦肩負教學訓練、培育後進之責。除輪訓之住院醫師外，亦有不少來自各醫學院之莘莘學子前來學習訓練。腎臟科由於教學風氣盛行，備受住院醫師與醫學生之肯定。然腎臟疾病之病生理機制複雜，對年輕醫師與醫學生而言，腎臟醫學常被認為是一門困難且艱深的學科。有感於此，北榮腎臟科於2016年特將腎臟科常見的臨床主題編纂為「腎臟醫學臨床技能手冊」一書，以各常見臨床主題為主幹，深入淺出，作為初入門學習臨床腎臟醫學之參考讀物。除可讓實習醫學生乃至於住院醫師都能有所增進腎臟學基礎知識，在面對實際臨床問題時更能據此進行明確判斷與合宜治療。七年來，此書贈與科內之輪訓住院醫師與醫學生閱讀，頗受肯定與讚賞，顯見此書之簡明扼要與實用性。

然而醫學知識日新月異，這七年來許多新的臨床試驗、臨床指引漸次更迭，亦有眾多新穎藥物相繼開發，書中內容及知識確實有更新必要。在內科部主任唐德成教授的支持、指導與鼓勵下，一年前偕同曾偉誠醫師開始籌備「腎臟醫學臨床技能手冊」之更新與再版，經過多位腎臟科醫師傾力修改及臨床經驗豐富的資深腎臟學老師校閱，使得「腎臟醫學臨床技能手冊」一書之改版得以順利付梓，甚是感激。

改版後的「腎臟醫學臨床技能手冊第二版」除更新原本各篇內容外，亦增加更多精美圖表解說，使讀者在閱讀理解上更容易、更有效率。再版內容遵循最新臨床指引撰寫，更加貼近讀者需求。並附上延伸閱讀資料，增廣及加強知識的深度和廣度，增添本書的可讀性，達到更完整的學習成效。

最後仍要由衷感謝參與文章及內容改版的所有腎臟科專科醫師及資深師長們，在繁忙臨床服務及研究教學之餘，撥冗齊心戮力參與本書改版，實屬不易。本書此次改版，即便已盡力修訂，仍難免有疏漏與不足之處，屆時亦請先進海涵與見諒，並不吝賜教，多予指導。

主編　林志慶　教授
臺北榮民總醫院腎臟科　主任
2023 年 4 月 28 日

目錄

序／林志慶 i

Chapter 1.　History Taking and Physical Examination ／周以新、歐朔銘 1

Chapter 2.　Problem-Oriented Differential Diagnosis of Common Symptoms and Signs in Nephrology ／胡譯安、莊喬琳 7

Chapter 3.　Acid-Base Disorders ／李景伯、林志慶 15

Chapter 4.　Sodium and Potassium ／牛志遠、曾偉誠 29

Chapter 5.　Laboratory Assessment of Renal Function by Blood and Urine ／李宗翰、蔡明村 53

Chapter 6.　Imaging: Diagnostic Characteristics of Common Kidney Diseases ／蔡友蓮、曾偉誠、沈書慧 65

Chapter 7.　Clinical Pharmacology ／王宗悅、楊智宇 85

Chapter 8.　Common Problems in Hemodialysis Patients ／陳紀瑜、林堯彬 95

Chapter 9.　Common Problems in Peritoneal Dialysis Patients ／陳範宇、陳進陽 111

Chapter 10.　Common Problems in Patients with Renal Transplant ／楊晴涵、吳采虹 133

Chapter 11.　Common Problems in Patients with Acute Kidney Injury ／何揚、李國華、唐德成 147

Chapter 12.　Diabetic Kidney Disease ／馬皓瑋、王植諄、黎思源 161

Chapter 1

History Taking and Physical Examination

周以新
臺北市立聯合醫院中興院區腎臟科
歐朔銘
臺北榮民總醫院腎臟科

正確的病史詢問與理學檢查是建立良好的醫病關係和提供有效的臨床思考方向。本章簡要地介紹腎臟學科相關之病史詢問與理學檢查之技巧，詳細的內容請參閱其他相關章節。

一、病史詢問

（一）基本資料 (Identifying Data)

病患的年齡、性別、種族及職業對於評估疾病很有幫助。例如，肉眼性血尿 (gross hematuria) 在年輕女性中最常見的原因是泌尿道感染。老年人若發現血尿，需藉由適當的檢查排除惡性疾病的可能性。美國非洲裔比美國白人具有更高之慢性腎臟病 (chronic kidney disease, CKD) 的盛行率。

（二）主訴 (Chief Complaint)

主訴能夠幫助醫療人員了解病人求診的主要目的及其症狀。此部分盡量以病人的語言記錄，例如：「我早上起來眼睛和臉浮腫」或「我腰痛，是不是腰子有問題」。CKD 早期，大部分病人沒有任何症狀，常為其他醫師於例行性檢查發現腎功能異常而轉診至腎臟科門診處理，常見與腎臟科相關的症狀，包含血尿、蛋白尿、頻尿、寡尿、夜尿、水腫、解尿疼痛、高血壓、疲倦、噁心、嘔吐等，皆必須詳加詢問。

（三）現在病史 (Present Illness)

這部分的病史應該依時序排列，完整描述症狀發生的時間、情況、表現形式和任何相關的治療。症狀的描述應包含：1. 位置 (**l**ocation)；2. 型態 (**q**uality)；3. 嚴重度 (**q**uantity)；4. 時間 (timing)，包含發作開始的時間、持續的時間和頻率 (**o**nset, duration, and frequency)；5. 誘發因素 (**p**recipitating factors)；6. 加劇和緩解因素 (**e**xaggerating and **r**elieving factors)；7. 伴隨的症狀 (**a**ssociated manifestations)。這幾個特性可以口訣「LQQOPERA」來幫助記憶。

(1) 血尿的外觀是可樂色 (cola-colored) 或烟色 (smoky) 通常是來自腎絲球 (glomerular) 出血。肉眼性血尿伴隨血塊通常為下泌尿道出血所致。以肉眼性血尿而言，出血在排尿的哪個階段最為明顯對於診斷很有幫助。排尿開始時的血尿表示源自尿道的出血，而結束時的血尿表示出血可能源自膀胱頸或前列腺病變。其他伴隨症狀亦是病史詢問的重點。絞痛 (colicky pain)，特別是輻射到會陰部，表示結石、血塊或脫落的腎乳頭 (renal papilla) 造成輸尿管阻塞。此外，激烈運動也可能導致血尿。

(2) 腎炎症候群 (nephritic syndrome) 的典型特徵是腎絲球血尿及活性的尿液沉渣，如 dysmorphic red blood cells (RBCs)、RBC casts、white blood cells (WBCs) 及 WBC casts，通常會伴隨腎絲球過濾率下降，以及不同程度的高血壓、寡尿及水腫。上呼吸道感染往往會加重 A 型免疫球蛋白腎病 (immunoglobulin A nephropathy)，並同時伴隨肉眼性血尿的發生 (synpharyngitic hematuria)。這與鏈球菌感染後腎絲球腎炎 (poststreptococcal glomerulonephritis) 的臨床表現不同，其血尿發生於感染後 (postpharyngitic hematuria) 的 2 至 6 週。紅斑性狼瘡 (systemic lupus erythematosus, SLE) 造成的腎炎症候群可能會伴隨發燒、皮疹及關節疼痛等症狀。

(3) 腎病症候群 (nephrotic syndrome) 包含主要五個臨床表現：A. 蛋白尿流失大於每日 3–3.5 g、B. 血清白蛋白低於 3 gm/dL、C. 水腫、D. 高血脂症和 E. 脂尿症。某些病人會描述尿液產生許多不會馬上化開的泡沫。腎病症候群可以是原發的 (idiopathic)，也可以是其他系統性疾病產生的併發症。糖尿病是系統性疾病中最常引發腎病症候群的原因。某些感染性疾病也是腎病症候群的原因，如病毒性肝炎、人類免疫缺乏病毒 (human immunodeficiency virus) 及梅毒等。

(4) 急性腎損傷 (acute kidney injury, AKI) 可藉由 RIFLE (risk, injury, failure, loss, end-stage)、AKIN (AKI Network) 或 KDIGO (Kidney Disease Improving Global Outcomes) 診斷準則加以定義。然而，在某些情況之下，近期相對的血清肌酸酐濃度無法順利獲得。特殊的病史特徵可將 AKI 的原因做適當的分類，例如：無尿（阻塞性尿路病變）；腸胃道出血、燒燙傷、腹瀉或脫水等（腎前性）；腎毒性藥物、缺血時間過長、敗血症、急性腎絲球腎炎或急性間質性腎炎等（腎因性）。若病患近期內接受過介入性處置，則 AKI 可能是因為顯影劑或是 atheroembolic disease 所致。若伴隨著發燒、關節痛、鼻竇炎及咳血的症狀，腎絲球腎炎便可能是 AKI 的原因。

(5) CKD 持續的時間和進展的速度對於疾病的治療對策很重要；是否就腎臟替代療法提出過相關的討論，必須於病歷紀錄載明清楚。CKD 的臨床表現和併發症可影響身體的每一個器官。因此，醫師應盡可能獲得任何可用的實驗室數據、腎臟切片報告和影像檢查的結果，增進病況的評估以減緩腎功能惡化的速度以及減少心血管疾病的風險。

（四）過去病史 (Past History)

1. 內科病史 (medical)：如糖尿病、高血壓、SLE、B 型肝炎、C 型肝炎、硬皮症 (scleroderma) 或血管炎等皆是 CKD 的可能病因。冠狀動脈疾病是 CKD 患者最重要的血管併發症。CKD 為 AKI 發生的相關危險因子。心衰竭與肝硬化會造成有效動脈內容積 (effective circulating volume) 不足，也會造成 AKI。此外，SLE 及各種形式的 systemic amyloidosis

會造成腎病症候群。腫瘤性疾病，包含各種 solid malignancies、淋巴瘤及白血病等也會造成腎病症候群。
2. 外科病史 (surgical)：紀錄手術的日期及種類，如泌尿系統的惡性疾病或體外震波碎石術等。
3. 婦產科病史 (obstetric and gynecologic)：伴隨著月經週期性的肉眼性血尿很可能是因為泌尿道子宮內膜異位症 (endometriosis) 所造成。

（五）家族史 (Family History)

單基因家族性腎臟疾病 (monogenic) 包含多囊性腎病 (polycystic kidney disease)、Alport's disease 和 Fabry's disease 等。大腦動脈瘤為多囊性腎病最致命的腎外併發症，常好發於家族成員中，於詢問家族史時須特別留意。多基因家族性疾病包含糖尿病、高血壓、肥胖、高脂血症和心血管疾病等。某些腎炎症候群及腎病症候群也會以家族性疾病的形式表現。

（六）個人和社會史 (Personal and Social History)

1. 藥物 (medications)：除了現在及過去所使用的藥物之外，還需包含非處方藥物及中草藥等，這些藥物除了可能具有腎毒性之外,有些也是造成腎病症候群的原因。具有腎毒性的藥物應特別註明，如 calcineurin inhibitor、lithium、pamidronate、cisplatin 和許多止痛藥等。Non-steroidal anti-inflammatory drugs (NSAIDs)、angiotensin converting enzyme inhibitor 和 angiotensin-II receptor blocker 併用利尿劑時，有可能會造成 AKI。會造成腎病症候群的藥物有 NSAIDs、penicillamine 及某些抗生素等。接受抗凝血劑治療可造成泌尿系統出血。
2. 長期暴露於抽菸、有機染料（如苯胺，aniline）等環境、接受某些化療藥物（如 cyclophosphamide）以及骨盆腔放射線治療，這些狀況會增加泌尿上皮癌的危險，有時會以血尿為初始的表現。

（七）系統回顧 (Review of Systems)

這一部分的目的在於確認是否存在某些被患者所忽略的問題。對於主訴具有正向 (pertinent positives) 或反向 (pertinent negatives) 證據的問題，可將這部分的紀錄移轉到現在病史。當患者於進行系統回顧時回想起患有那些疾病，也可以將這些疾病補充記錄在現在病史或過去病史中。
1. 一般 (general)：近期體重變化，尿毒性口臭 (uremic fetor)，疲倦，無力或發燒。
2. 皮膚：紅疹，搔癢或皮膚顏色改變。

3. 頭、眼、耳、鼻、喉 (head, ear, eyes, nose, throat, HEENT)：糖尿病及高血壓常造成 CKD 患者眼科的併發症。Alport's disease 患者可能會有聽力喪失與水晶體的異常。視力模糊或鼻竇發炎可能是由續發性腎絲球腎炎所造成。
4. 呼吸系統：咳血可能是血管炎或 anti-glomerular basement membrane disease (anti-GBM) 所造成。
5. 心血管系統：休息、運動時胸痛或呼吸困難。
6. 消化系統：食慾狀況，味覺改變，厭食，噁心，嘔吐，腹痛，腹瀉，腹脹。
7. 泌尿系統：寡尿，多尿，頻尿，夜尿，延遲排尿 (hesitancy)，失禁，尿路感染，背痛，腰痛，骨盆痛，腎結石，血尿。
8. 周邊血管系統：間歇性跛行，下肢壞疽，小腿、足部腫脹。
9. 肌肉骨骼系統：肌肉痙攣 (muscle cramps)，肌肉萎縮，骨骼及關節痛，痛風。
10. 神經系統：記憶力、情緒和睡眠模式的改變，不自主運動。

二、理學檢查

(一) 腎臟 (Kidneys)

　　腎臟的位置位於第 12 肋骨和脊椎的夾角交界處，又稱為肋脊角 (costovertebral angle, CV angle)。腎臟所處的高度約在 T11–L3 之間，長度約為 9–12 cm，寬度約為 5–6 cm，厚度約為 3–4 cm。而因為肝臟的關係，右腎的位置會比左腎略低。

　　腎臟位於身體較深處，因此在正常情況下很難觸摸的到，往往需要比肝臟或脾臟進行更深部的觸診，當腎臟急性發炎或是有腫瘤形成的時候，腎臟可能會變大，此時可以透過觸診來檢查。觸診腎臟時，我們可以要求病人深呼吸，並在病人深呼吸時，將一隻手在第 12 肋下緣位置將腎臟往上方推，另一隻手再從上方深壓，以觸摸位於較深處的腎臟，觸摸時可檢查是否有腎臟腫大 (kidney enlargements) 或出現腎臟腫塊 (kidney mass) 的情形。

(二) 肋脊角檢查 (CV Angle Examination)

　　當病患因為有腎炎，腎盂腎炎，腎結石，腎周圍膿瘍等情形，而使腎臟夾膜撐大 (distended renal capsule) 會引起疼痛，這樣的疼痛屬於持續且悶悶的腰痛 (dull constant flank pain)，痛感約位於 T11–L2 的 spinal cords level，並沿著 subcostal region 往肚臍方向傳遞，此時病患敲擊痛 (knocking pain) 會呈現陽性反應。敲擊痛檢查方式為請病人坐直，把一支手放在 CV angle 上，另一手握拳往下輕敲，看病患是否有痛感。

（三）腎動脈 (Renal Artery)

腎動脈 (renal arteries) 為由腹主動脈垂直左右分出，位置約在劍突 (xiphoid process) 到肚臍 (umbilicus) 連線的中點右邊或左邊 3–4cm 處，我們可以利用聽診的方式於 renal artery 上方檢查是否有聽到雜音 (bruit)，若有則表示可能有腎動脈狹窄 (renal artery stenosis) 的情形，這是因為血流流經狹窄的動脈所產生的聲音，一部分是亂流所引起，而另一部分則是由動脈壁振動引起的。

（四）膀胱 (Bladder)

正常情況下，膀胱是無法觸摸的，但是當膀胱脹尿至 150 mL 時可被觸摸到。若是恥骨上區域 (suprapubic area) 出現疼痛 (tenderness) 則表示病患可能有膀胱炎 (cystitis) 的情形。必須注意的是，理學檢查時利用叩診 (percussion) 的方式，可以比觸診 (palpation) 更容易確認膀胱真正的位置。

延伸閱讀文獻

Bickley LS, Szilagyi PG. Overview: physical examination and history taking. In: Bickley LS, Szilagyi PG, eds. *Bates' Guide to Physical Examination and History Taking*. 11th ed. Philadelphia, PA: Lippincott Williams and Wilkins; 2012:3-13.

Sakhaee K, Moe OW. Urolithiasis. In: Yu ASL, Chertow G, Luyckx V, Marsden P, Skorecki K, Taal M, eds. *Brenner and Rector's The Kidney*. 11th ed. Philadelphia, PA: Elsevier; 2020:1277-1326.

Waikar SS, Bonventre JV. Disorders of the kidney and urinary tract. In: Kasper DL, Fauci AS, Hauser SL, Longo DL, Jameson JL, Loscalzo J, eds. *Harrison's Principles of Internal Medicine*. 19th ed. New York, NY: McGraw Hill Education; 2015:1799-1874.

Chapter 2

Problem-Oriented Differential Diagnosis of Common Symptoms and Signs in Nephrology

胡譯安
臺北榮民總醫院腎臟科
莊喬琳
臺北榮民總醫院腎臟科

一、Hematuria

尿液經低速離心沉澱後，取沉澱物在四百倍之高倍鏡視野 (high power field, HPF) 下觀察，若紅血球 (red blood cells, RBC) 數目為 3 至 5 個以上 (≥ 3–5 RBC/HPF)，即為血尿。

（一）Types of Hematuria

1. 肉眼性血尿：肉眼可見紅色、粉紅、或棕色尿液。
2. 顯微性血尿：尿液顏色正常（鑑別診斷流程詳參 Figure 2-1）。

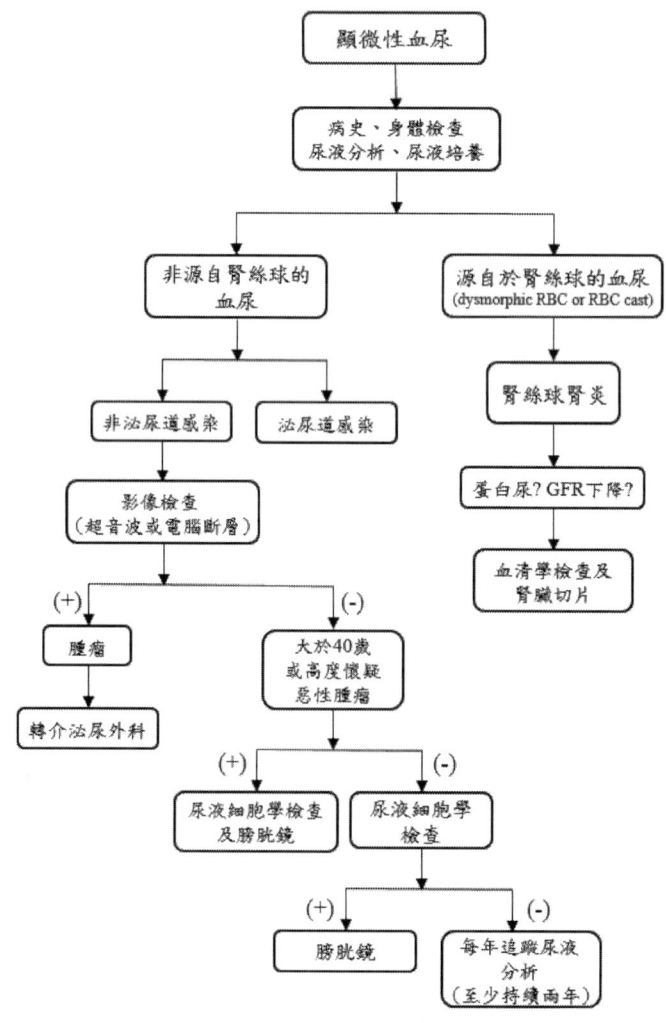

Figure 2-1. 顯微性血尿診斷流程

（二）Origin of Hematuria

1. Non-Glomerular Hematuria

非源自腎絲球的血尿，多因泌尿道結石、感染、腫瘤、或外傷出血造成 (Table 2-1)。

2. Glomerular Hematuria

源自於腎絲球的血尿，多為腎絲球疾病造成。特徵為 dysmorphic RBCs，常伴隨有蛋白尿 (> 0.5 g/day) (Table 2-2)。

Table 2-1. 非源自腎絲球的血尿常見的原因

位置	病因
上泌尿道	尿路結石
	腎盂腎炎
	腎細胞癌
	泌尿道上皮細胞癌
	腎臟水腫
	外傷
下泌尿道	膀胱炎
	攝護腺肥大
	泌尿道上皮細胞癌
	外傷
	藥物 (e.g., warfarin)

Table 2-2. 腎絲球的血尿常見的原因

分類	疾病
增生性腎絲球腎炎	A 型免疫球蛋白腎病變
	全身性血管炎
	感染後腎絲球腎炎
	膜增生性腎絲球腎炎
	狼瘡腎炎
	快速進行性腎炎
	混合性冷凝球蛋白血症
非增生性腎絲球腎炎	局部節段性腎絲球硬化症
	膜性腎病變
家族性腎絲球疾病	薄腎絲球基底膜疾病
	亞伯氏症候群 (Alport's syndrome)

二、Edema

因組織間隙或循環系統有過多的液體堆積，造成局部肢體或全身性腫脹（各種水腫原因詳參 Table 2-3，診斷流程詳參 Figure 2-2）。

（一）Pathophysiology

1. Increased capillary hydrostatic pressure.
2. Increased capillary permeability.
3. Reduced capillary osmotic pressure.
4. Lymphatic obstruction.
5. Retention of salt and water.

（二）Distribution of Edema

1. 局部水腫：單側或單一肢體腫脹，多源自靜脈或淋巴管循環阻塞。
2. 全身性水腫：全身對稱性腫脹，多源自肝、心、腎、荷爾蒙異常。

Table 2-3. 水腫常見的原因

病生理機轉	病因
微血管靜水壓上升	心衰竭
	腎衰竭
	肝硬化
	靜脈阻塞
微血管通透性上升	燒燙傷
	過敏反應
	感染、敗血症
滲透壓下降	腎病症候群
	肝硬化
	營養不良
	吸收不良
淋巴回流受阻	淋巴絲蟲病
	淋巴切除
	腫瘤造成之淋巴結腫大
其他	甲狀腺功能低下
	不明原因水腫

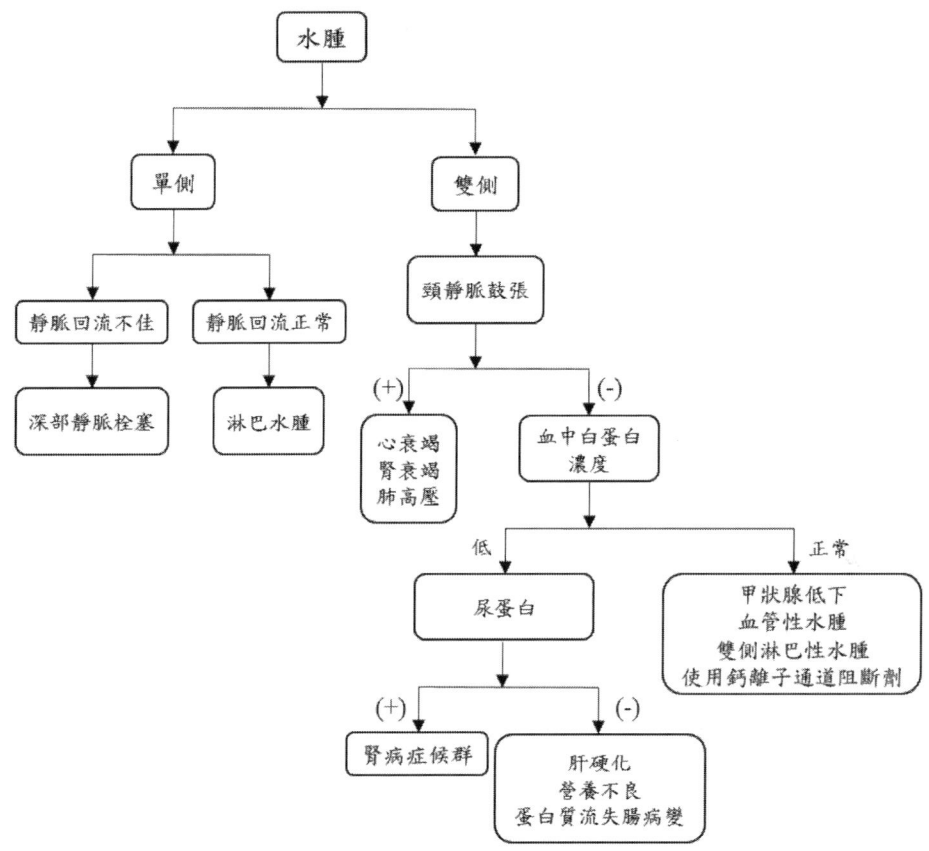

Figure 2-2. 水腫診斷流程

（三）Types of Edema

1. Pitting edema.（用手指加壓會有凹陷，稍後才能平復）
2. Non-pitting edema.（淋巴液堆積，水腫皮膚變硬，不易出現凹陷）

三、Proteinuria

健康成年人每天尿中蛋白質排出量應少於 150 mg，若多於 150 mg 就稱為蛋白尿。如果每天尿蛋白量超過 3.5 g，稱為腎病症候群。

（一）Measurement

1. 尿液試紙（僅能偵測尿中的白蛋白）(Table 2-4)。

Table 2-4. Urine dipstick proteinuria

Dipstick test	Proteinuria
Trace	≒ 10–20 mg/dL
1+	≒ 30 mg/dL
2+	≒ 100 mg/dL
3+	≒ 300 mg/dL
4+	> 1 g/dL

2. 利用單次尿液的蛋白質／肌酸酐比值評估 24 小時尿蛋白排出量 (spot urine protein/creatinine ratio ≒ g of 24-hr proteinuria)。
3. 收集 24 小時的尿液精確測量尿蛋白排出量。

（二）Type of Proteinuria

1. 暫時性蛋白尿：發燒或劇烈運動所致。
2. 姿勢性蛋白尿：直立時才出現蛋白尿（躺著時沒有），只發生於年輕人，通常 20 歲以後消失。
3. 持續性蛋白尿：因腎臟疾病或全身性疾病造成。

（三）Etiology of Proteinuria

蛋白尿常見原因見 Table 2-5，診斷流程見 Figure 2-3。

1. Glomerular: Protein loss due to glomerulonephritis (> 3.5 g/day).
2. Tubular: Decreased tubular reabsorption of low molecular weight protein due to tubular or interstitial disease (1–2 g/day).
3. Overflow: Increased production of monoclonal immunoglobulin.

四、Flank Pain

許多人認為腰部疼痛是腎臟病引起，事實上，大部分的腎臟病是不會疼痛的，腎臟病主要的表現是蛋白尿和水腫。會引起腰痛的腎臟疾病主要是腎結石、急性腎盂腎炎或腎血管栓塞 (Table 2-6)。

Table 2-5. 蛋白尿常見的原因

種類	病因
原發性腎絲球病變	微小病變腎病
	原發性膜性腎小球腎炎
	局部節段性腎絲球硬化症
	膜增生性腎絲球腎炎
	A 型免疫球蛋白腎病變
次發性腎絲球病變	糖尿病
	高血壓性腎硬化
	狼瘡腎炎
	澱粉樣蛋白疾病
	感染（例如：HIV、HBV、HCV、梅毒、心內膜炎）
	腫瘤
	藥物（例如：海洛因、非類固醇類止痛藥、抗生素）
	腎小管間質性疾病
	范康尼氏症候群 (Fanconi syndrome)
	鐮刀型紅血球疾病
	重金屬
	急性過敏性間質腎炎
製造過多	多發性骨髓瘤

Abbreviations: HBV, hepatitis B virus; HCV, hepatitis C virus; HIV, human immunodeficiency virus.

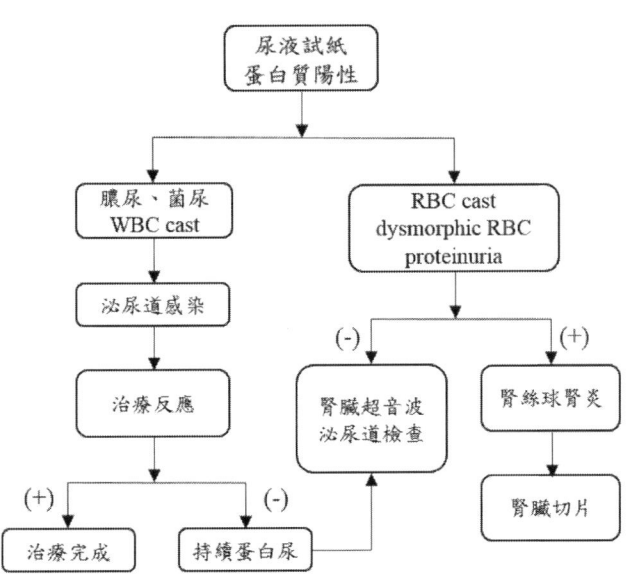

Figure 2-3. 蛋白尿診斷流程

Abbreviations: RBC, red blood cells; WBC, white blood cells.

Table 2-6. 腰痛常見的原因

種類	病因
腎因性	尿路結石
	阻塞性尿路疾病
	腎絲球腎炎或腎膿
	腎靜脈栓塞
	腎梗塞
非腎因性	骨骼肌肉疼痛
	帶狀皰疹
	肋膜炎或肺炎
	後腹腔疾病（例如：淋巴癌、轉移性腫瘤）
	婦產科疾病（例如：異位妊娠、骨盆腔炎症）
	腹主動脈瘤
	髂腰肌膿瘍
	脊神經根炎

延伸閱讀文獻

Davis R, Jones JS, Barocas DA, et al; American Urological Association. Diagnosis, evaluation and follow-up of asymptomatic microhematuria (AMH) in adults: AUA guideline. *J Urol*. 2012;188(6 Suppl):2473-2481. doi:10.1016/j.juro.2012.09.078

Emmett M, Fenves AZ, Schwartz JC. Approach to the patient with kidney disease. In: Taal MW, Chertow GM, Marsden PA, Skorecki K, Yu ASL, Brenner BM, eds. *Brenner and Rector's the Kidney*. 9th ed. Philadelphia, PA: Elsevier; 2011:844-867.

Chapter 3
Acid-Base Disorders

李景伯
台北榮民總醫院腎臟科
林志慶
台北榮民總醫院腎臟科

一、Introduction

人體酸鹼恆定 (pH within 7.35–7.45) 主要由兩大部分完成，一是血中的酸鹼中和系統，二則是由肺與腎進行的 CO_2 排除與 HCO_3^- 的再生、排出／再吸收。

（一）酸鹼中和系統與 Henderson–Hasselbalch Equation

人體內血中的酸鹼需維持恆定，才能確保各種蛋白及酵素之生理活性正常。酸（可釋出 H^+ 者）與酸根（可接受 H^+ 者，也就是共軛鹼）之間的平衡連動關係，由以下 Henderson–Hasselbalch equation 化學方程式一以貫之：

$$pH = pK_a + \log\left(\frac{[A^-]}{[HA]}\right)$$

pH：酸鹼值，K_a：解離常數，[HA]：酸的莫耳濃度，$[A^-]$：共軛鹼的莫耳濃度

碳酸氫根 (HCO_3^-) 是人體內血中最主要可做為緩衝的決定性鹼基，所以要了解血中 pH 的動態變化，可將上列公式改寫如下：

$$pH = pK_a(H_2CO_3) + \log\left(\frac{[HCO_3^-]}{[H_2CO_3]}\right)$$

pH：酸鹼值，K_a：H_2CO_3 的解離常數，$[H_2CO_3]$：碳酸的莫耳濃度，$[HCO_3^-]$：碳酸氫根的莫耳濃度。

血中碳酸與血中 CO_2 的分壓和溶解係數 (k_H, Henry constant) 有相關如下：

$$[H_2CO_3] = k_{HCO_2} \times pCO_2$$

而 k_{HCO_2} 約是 0.0307 mmol/(L-torr)；$pK_a(H_2CO_3)$：碳酸解離常數之負 $\log_{10}$ 值，約是 6.1，所以可將上列公式代換如下：

$$pH = 6.1 + \log\left(\frac{[HCO_3^-]}{0.03 \times pCO_2}\right)$$

由上述公式可知，H_2CO_3 的 pK_a 遠小於正常 pH 值 7.4，所以絕大多數的血中 H_2CO_3 是以 HCO_3^- 的型態留存，作為細胞外液中最重要的緩衝系統，藉由調控 HCO_3^- 的濃度與 CO_2 的清除，人體達成血中的酸鹼恆定。

（二）Normal Value and Normal Range

完整評估血液酸鹼狀態至少需要抽檢動脈血液氣體分析 (arterial blood gas, ABG) 或靜脈血液氣體分析 (venous blood gas, VBG)，兩者正常值及正常範圍如 Table 3-1：

Table 3-1. Normal values of arterial/venous blood gas data

Arterial blood	Mean	Range
pH	7.4	7.36 to 7.44
$[H^+]$, nM	40	36 to 44
PCO_2, mmHg	40	36 to 44
$[HCO_3^-]$, mM	24	22 to 26
Base excess	0	−2 to +2
Venous blood	Mean	Range
pH	7.38	7.34 to 7.42
$[H^+]$, nM	42	38 to 46
PCO_2, mmHg	46	42 to 50
CO_2 total, mM	26	23 to 30

各種酸鹼不平衡的對應變化可詳參 Table 3-2：

Table 3-2. Changes of arterial blood gas data in metabolic acidosis and metabolic alkalosis

	Metabolic acidosis	Metabolic alkalosis	Respiratory acidosis	Respiratory alkalosis
pH	< 7.35	> 7.45	< 7.35	> 7.45
HCO_3^-	< 22	> 26	Acute: ↑ 0.1 × ΔPCO$_2$ Chronic: ↑ 0.3 × ΔPCO$_2$	Acute: ↓ 0.2 × ΔPCO$_2$ Chronic: ↓ 0.4–0.5 × ΔPCO$_2$
PCO_2	↓ 1.2–1.3 × Δ$[HCO_3^-]$	↑ 0.6–0.7 × Δ$[HCO_3^-]$	> 45	< 35
Time to reach compensation	12–24 hours	24–36 hours	Acute < 10 min Chronic: 3–4 days	Acute < 10 min Chronic: 2–3 days
Limit of compensation	PCO_2 ≥ 15 mmHg	PCO_2 ≤ 55 mmHg	$[HCO_3^-]$ Acute: 38 mM Chronic: 45 mM	$[HCO_3^-]$ Acute: 18 mM Chronic: 15 mM

（三）Anion Gap (AG)

在評估體內血液酸鹼狀態時，除了以血中 pH 值初步判定是酸抑或鹼之外，倘若有代謝性酸血症時，往往需進一步分析是 high AG metabolic acidosis 還是 normal AG acidosis？那到底什麼是 AG 呢？

如 Figure 3-1 中的 A 所示，血中的陽離子和陰離子當量相等，如此才可維持血液的電中性平衡。而血中的陽離子主要有 Na^+、K^+、Ca^{2+}、Mg^{2+}，而陰離子主要有 Cl^-、HCO_3^-、$PO_4^{3-}/HPO_4^{2-}/H_2PO_4^-$、$SO_4^{2-}$、其他的有機酸、protein 等等。陽離子和陰離子的平衡可以下列等式簡單表示：

$$[Na^+] + [K^+] + [Ca^{2+}] + [Mg^{2+}] + [\text{Unmeasured cations}]$$
$$= [HCO_3^-] + [Cl^-] + [\text{Albumin (Alb)}] + [\text{Unmeasured anions}]$$

將上式整理移位後可以得到：

$$[AG] = [\text{Unmeasured anions}] - [\text{Unmeasured cations}]$$
$$= [Na^+] + [K^+] + [Ca^{2+}] + [Mg^{2+}] - [HCO_3^-] - [Cl^-] - [Alb]$$

然後從 Figure3-1 中的 A 可知，$[Ca^{2+}]$、$[Mg^{2+}]$ 僅占主要陽離子約 5% 且一般變化相對較小，再者早年因為檢驗不便，主要化驗的陽離子為 Na^+、K^+，Alb 也不見的能測，所以也可將上列公式改寫為：

$$[Na^+] + [K^+] - [HCO_3^-] - [Cl^-] = [AG] = [\text{Unmeasured anions}] - [\text{Unmeasured cations}]$$

如 Figure3-1 中的 B 及 C 所示：

$$AG = [Na^+] + [K^+] - [HCO_3^-] - [Cl^-] = 15$$
或者
$$AG = [Na^+] - [HCO_3^-] - [Cl^-] = 10$$

然而，酸血症時常會造成 K 離子的 transcellular shift，臨床上以 Figure 3-1 中的 C 的公式為主：

$$AG = [Na^+] - [HCO_3^-] - [Cl^-] = 10\text{–}12 \text{ (mmol/L)}$$

此外，以臺灣現今醫療水準發達，基本上沒有不測定 Alb 的時空背景，因此 AG 值也需要以 Alb (g/dL) × 2.5 校正。AG 變化及可能原因如 Table 3-3。

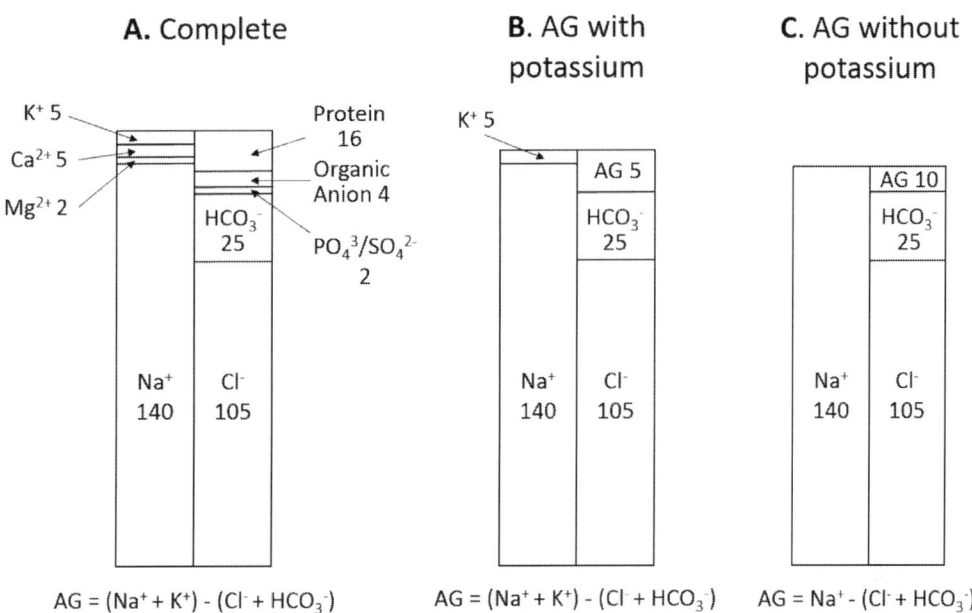

Figure 3-1. Ionic balance in serum (unit: mmol/L)

AG, anion gap.

Table 3-3. Causes of AG change

Change of AG	Change of blood chemistry
AG ↑	Alb ↑
	Unmeasured anions (organic acids, phosphates, sulfates) ↑
	Uremia
	Unmeasured cations (Ca^{2+}, Mg^{2+}) ↓
AG ↓	Alb ↓
	Unmeasured cations（Ca^{2+}, Mg^{2+}, K^+, Li^+ 或 immunoglobulin 如 IgG）↑
	bromide ↑

Abbreviations: AG, anion gap; Alb, albumin.

（四）Approach to Metabolic Acidosis

代謝性酸中毒到底要如何進行鑑別診斷呢？

1. 第零步：確認病人的病史與臨床狀況

例如呼吸器的病人沒調設定不會有額外的代償，嚴重脫水／低血鉀的病人會混有代謝性鹼血症。

Chapter 3 Acid-Base Disorders

2. **第一步：驗算 [HCO$_3^-$] 的數值是否為真，有無過度偏差？**

    動脈血機測量錯誤（CO$_2$ 逸散、電阻測定錯算 pH 等）。

    (1) Calculated [HCO$_3^-$] = 24 × PCO$_2$ / [H$^+$] (mM)。

    (2) Measured [HCO$_3^-$] – calculated [HCO$_3^-$] 應該要在 ± 3 之間。

3. **第二步：計算 AG**

    詳見前段（三）Anion Gap (AG)。

    AG = [Na$^+$] – [Cl$^-$] – [HCO$_3^-$] = 10 ± 2（血中 [Alb] = 4.5 g/dL 的狀況下）

    校正：血中 [Alb] 每下降 1 g/dL，AG 會下降 2.5 mEq/L

4. **第三步：確認是否為 High AG Metabolic Acidosis，做進一步鑑別診斷**

    詳見下段二、High AG Metabolic Acidosis。

5. **第四步：確認是否為 Normal AG Metabolic Acidosis，做進一步鑑別診斷**

    詳見下段三、Normal AG Metabolic Acidosis。

6. **第五步：呼吸代償是否恰當？**

    (1) PCO$_2$ 的代償極限：10–15 mmHg。

    (2) 計算合理代償 PCO$_2$ 的應有值。

    PCO$_2$ = 1.5 × [HCO$_3^-$] + 8 ± 2

    PCO$_2$ = [HCO$_3^-$] + 15

    PCO$_2$ = ABG 的 pH 值小數點後兩位 (e.g., PCO$_2$ = 25 when pH = 7.25)

7. **第六步：是否合併有其他酸中毒或鹼中毒？**

    計算「Delta/Delta ratio, Δ/Δ」值，詳見下段二、High AG Metabolic Acidosis

二、High AG Metabolic Acidosis

代謝性酸血症合併 AG 過高，就是「high AG metabolic acidosis」，通常代表多出新的酸根。反之，如果有代謝性酸血症但是 AG 數值正常，則為「normal AG metabolic acidosis」。然而，臨床上遇到的情況有時並不單純，代謝性酸血症可能會合併其他代謝性異常，此時應計算「AG 變化值」和「HCO$_3$ 變化值」兩者之間的比值，也就是「Delta/Delta ratio (Δ/Δ)」：

$$\Delta/\Delta = \Delta AG / \Delta HCO_3^-$$
$$= (\text{measured AG} - \text{calculated AG}) / (24 - \text{measured HCO}_3^-)$$
= 新多出的酸根 / 中和的鹼量 [由此可判斷代謝性酸血症受高 AG 酸的相關程度] (Table 3-4)

*血中中和系統一般認為由約 50% 的 HCO_3^-、35% hemoglobin 與 5% HPO_4^- 組成。

到底有哪些原因會造成 high AG metabolic acidosis 呢？以下口訣可供快速回憶，探詢可能造成 high AG metabolic acidosis 的原因：「A MUD PILES（一堆泥樁）」Table 3-5。

Table 3-4. Interpretation of Delta/Delta (Δ/Δ)

Change of Δ/Δ	Corresponding metabolic abnormalities
$\Delta/\Delta = 1{\sim}2$	Pure high AG metabolic acidosis
$\Delta/\Delta < 1$	High AG metabolic acidosis + normal AG metabolic acidosis
	Hyperchloremic metabolic acidosis
$\Delta/\Delta > 2$	High AG metabolic acidosis + Metabolic alkalosis / chronic respiratory acidosis

Abbreviation: AG, anion gap.

Table 3-5. High anion gap metabolic acidosis 各類病因的症狀學 (A MUD PILES)

疾病	症狀
Alcohol	詳見 Table 3-6
Methanol	詳見 Table 3-6
Uremia	噁心嘔吐、食慾不振、貧血及出血傾向、皮膚搔癢、高血壓、水腫、高血鉀症、高血磷症和低鈣血症等
Diabetic ketoacidosis	高血糖（> 250 mg/dL）、呼吸急促、呼氣中有水果味（丙酮）、噁心、嘔吐、腹痛、意識障礙、昏迷
Pyroglutamic acid	肝功能異常、肝炎
	可能由 Acetaminophen（最常見）、Vigabatrin、Flucloxacillin、Netilmicin 引起，Glycine 攝取不足也會造成 pyroglutamic acid 酸中毒（可能原因：敗血症、營養不良、懷孕、第二型糖尿病）
	可使用 N-acetylcysteine 治療
Isoniazid	抽搐、昏迷、肝功能異常、周邊神經病變
Lactic acidosis	疲倦嗜睡、全身無力、肌肉痠痛、呼吸困難、眩暈、意識障礙、血壓下降、心跳減慢、昏迷
Ethylene glycol	詳見 Table 3-6.
Salicylate (Aspirin)	詳見 Table 3-6.

各種不同造成 high AG metabolic acidosis 的原因要如何區分確診呢？可由合併之臨床症狀和徵兆進行鑑別診斷（參考 Table 3-5）。

如果是毒藥物所引起的 high AG metabolic acidosis，可進一步根據 AG 變化及 osmolal gap (OG) 變化做鑑別診斷，區分為以下幾類 (Table 3-6)：

$$\text{Serum OG} = \text{measured serum osmolality (Osm)} - \text{calculated serum Osm}$$
$$= \text{unmeasured cations/anions that provide Osm}$$

三、Normal AG Metabolic Acidosis

有代謝性酸血症但是 AG 數值正常，常見可分成腸胃／腎的鹼 HCO_3^- 流失、高氯負荷等，那又確切有哪些原因會造成 normal AG metabolic acidosis 呢？可以用 Table 3-7 口訣快速回憶，探討可能造成 normal AG metabolic acidosis 的原因：「USED CARPS（用過的車皮們）」。

各種不同造成 normal AG metabolic acidosis 的原因要如何區分確診呢？可由合併之臨床症狀和徵兆進行鑑別診斷（參考 Tables 3-7–9）：

四、Renal Tubular Acidosis (RTA)

（一）不論是 high AG metabolic acidosis 或是 normal AG acidosis，治療貴在矯正造成代謝性酸中毒的根本病因，而非一味地給予碳酸氫鈉補充。

（二）到底哪些病患需要給予鹼化劑治療呢？大部分情形並無共識或準則，但一般而言，「嚴重的（有症狀的）急性代謝性酸中毒合併 pH < 7.10」或可做為

Table 3-6. Differential diagnosis of intoxication related high AG metabolic acidosis

AG 變化	OG 變化	疾病	臨床症狀
↑	正常	Acetaminophen	肝功能異常、肝炎
		Salicylates	發燒、心跳過速、耳鳴；合併有呼吸性鹼中毒
↑	↑	Alcohol (ethanol)	酒臭味、意識改變、肝炎；同時合併有酮酸中毒、乳酸中毒和代謝性鹼中毒
		Methanol	意識變化改變、視力模糊、瞳孔放大、視乳突水腫
		Ethylene glycol	意識變化、心肺衰竭、低血鈣、尿中有草酸鈣結晶甚至因此急性腎傷害
		Propylene glycol	急性腎傷害
正常	↑	Isopropyl alcohol	意識改變、呼吸有水果味（丙酮）

Abbreviations: AG, anion gap; OG, osmol gap.

Table 3-7. Normal anion gap metabolic acidosis 各類病因的症狀學

疾病	病史、症狀
Uretero-enterostomy	手術病史
Small bowel fistula	手術病史、腹瀉、腹脹、腹痛、體重減輕
Excess Cl⁻ (NH$_4$Cl, CaCl$_2$)	給予大量含氯藥品補充
Expansion acidosis (saline infusion)	給予大量 normal saline 輸液（不含鹼基來源 [例如：乳酸]）
Diarrhea	腹瀉、虛弱無力、脫水
Drugs	藥物包括：NSAID, trimethoprim, ACEi, ARB, pentamidine, cyclosporine, K$^+$-sparing agent
Carbonic anhydrase inhibitors (acetazolamide)	眼睛不適、頭痛、胃腸道不適、腎結石、骨髓抑制
Adrenal insufficiency	疲倦嗜睡、無力、食慾不振、體重減輕、噁心、低血壓、皮膚色素沉著、低血鈉、高血鉀
Acid loads	Hippurate：吸食強力膠 Hyperalimentation：全靜脈營養
RTA	詳見 Table 3-8.
Pancreatic fistula	腹痛、胰臟炎、腹部外傷、體重減輕、腹水
Spironolactone	高血鉀、心律不整、男性女乳症、低血鈉

Abbreviations: ACEi, angiotensin converting enzyme inhibitors; ARB, angiotensin receptor blocker; NSAID, non-steroidal anti-inflammatory drug; RTA, renal tubular acidosis.

Table 3-8. Renal tubular acidosis 的實驗診斷與臨床鑑別診斷

實驗或臨床特徵	Proximal (Type II)	Classical distal (Type I)	Generalized distal (Type IV)
血鉀	低	低	高
尿的 pH 值	< 5.5	> 5.5	< 5.5 或 > 5.5
有無合併 Fanconi 病徵（尿糖、低血磷、低尿酸血症等）	有	無	無
FE$_{HCO3}$^{a}	> 10%–15%	< 5%	< 5%–10%
對於鹼化治療反應	最差	好	中等
合併之臨床特徵	Fanconi syndrome	腎鈣質沉積症 高球蛋白血症	腎功能不全

^{a}Fractional excretion of bicarbonate.

　　　給予鹼化劑治療之適應症。（糖尿病酮酸中毒例外，請依 American Diabetes Association guideline 為準。）

（三）給予碳酸氫鈉鹼化劑治療的劑量可用下列公式粗略估算：

Table 3-9. RTA 臨床特徵口訣

口訣	臨床特徵
一遠二近	Type 1 RTA = Distal RTA; Type 2 RTA = Proximal RTA
一石二軟	Type 1 RTA 容易有尿路結石、Type 2 RTA 容易有軟骨症
一尿不酸	Type 1 RTA 的尿液 pH 較高
四鉀朝天	Type 4 RTA 容易合併有高血鉀症

RTA, renal tubular acidosis.

HCO_3^- 缺乏總量 = HCO_3^- 分布係數 × 體重 × ([HCO_3^-] 目標值 − [HCO_3^-] 實際值)

HCO_3^- 分布係數 = 0.4 + 2.6 / [HCO_3^-]；[HCO_3^-] 目標值為 ≤ 0.6 × $PaCO_2$

例：[HCO_3^-] = 13 mEq/L 的狀況下，HCO_3^- 分布係數 = 0.4 + 2.6 / 13 = 0.4 + 0.2 = 0.6; 若 $PaCO_2$ = 33.3 mmHg, 則 [HCO_3^-] 目標值 ≤ 20 mEq/L

例：欲將一體重 70 kg 之代謝性酸中毒患者之血中 [HCO_3^-] 從 13 mEq/L 校正到 20 mEq/L，所需之 HCO_3^- 總量 = 0.6 × 70 kg × (20 − 13) = 294 mEq。目前臺灣通用之碳酸氫鈉針劑為濃度 7%，20 mL/amp 的劑型，每 amp 含 16.7 mEq，換算得知：總共需要 294 / 16.7 = 17.5 隻碳酸氫鈉靜脈注射液。

（四）由於碳酸氫鈉為高張、高鈉之靜脈注射製劑，所以治療時應避免高血鈉症的副作用產生。故給予大量時可考慮以 $NaHCO_3$ 4.5 amp (= 90 mL) + D5W 410 mL 製備成 [Na] = 150 mEq/L 的等張溶液給予靜脈輸注，避免造成高血鈉症。

（五）補充碳酸氫鈉之原則：
1. 治療目標：[HCO_3^-] ≤ 0.6 × PaO_2
   矯正速度：血中 [HCO_3^-] 上升應 < 2–4 mEq/L/hr
2. 如果沒有心臟或者腎臟疾病的狀況下，可在治療的前 3–4 個小時給予所需總量的 1/4–1/2。

五、Metabolic Alkalosis

（一）Pathophysiology

嚴重的代謝性鹼中毒可能會導致呼吸變緩、代償性的換氣量下降、全身抽筋、甚至心律不整。代謝性鹼中毒通常都會有兩個階段：第一個階段是「代謝性鹼中毒的產生」，第二個階段是「代謝性鹼中毒的維持因子（HCO_3^- 的排出減少）」，往往是兩者並存時才會產生顯著的代謝性鹼中毒：

1. **第一階段：代謝性鹼中毒的產生**
   (1) 體內酸的流失：嘔吐導致胃酸流失、低血鉀導致氫離子跑進細胞內、礦物性皮質素持續作用而使得腎臟排酸量上升。
   (2) 碳酸氫根的增加：服用或者靜脈給予過多碳酸氫鈉。

2. **第二階段：代謝性鹼中毒的維持因子（HCO_3^- 的排出減少）**
   (1) 腎絲球過濾率下降。
   (2) 體液不足導致血管內容積低下，進而誘發近端腎小管回收碳酸氫根增加。
   (3) 低血鉀症導致近端及遠端腎小管回收碳酸氫根增加。
   (4) 低血氯症。

（二）Clinical Approach to the Metabolic Alkalosis

如何找出代謝性鹼中毒的可能病因呢？Figure 3-2 流程圖可供參考：

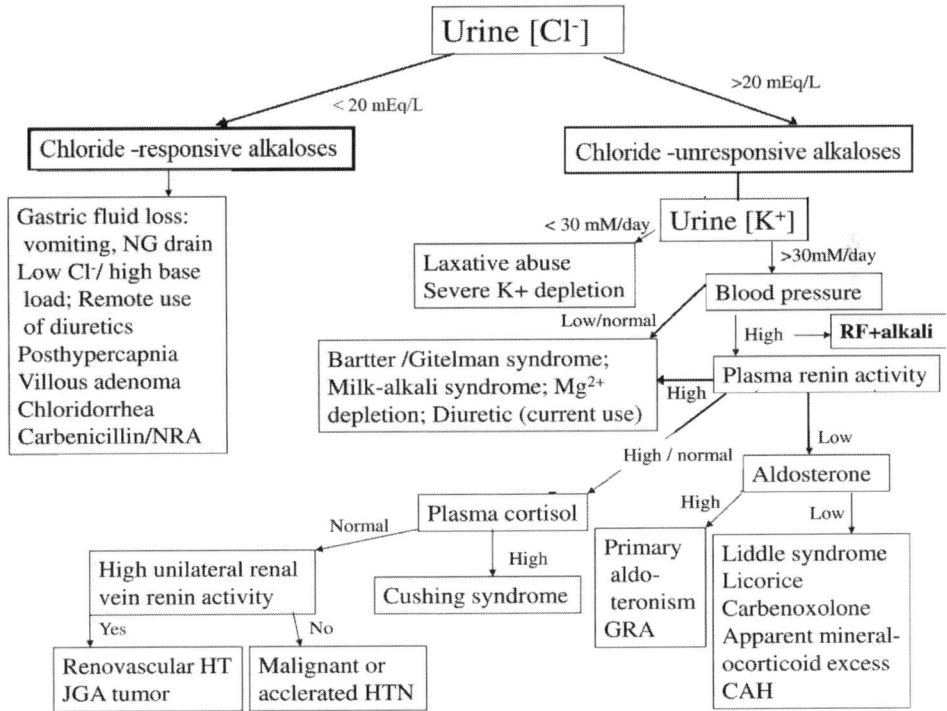

Figure 3-2. Diagnostic approach to metabolic alkalosis

Abbreviations: CAH, congenital adrenal hyperplasia; GRA, glucocorticoid remediable aldosteronism; HT, hypertension; HTN, hypertension; JGA, juxtaglomerular apparatus; NG, nasogastric; NRA, non-reabsorbable anion; RF, rheumatoid factor.

檢驗尿生化數值，其變化也可協助我們進行鑑別診斷（參考 Table 3-10）。

Table 3-10. Urine chemistry data and associated metabolic alkalosis disorder

	U [Na$^+$]	U [K$^+$]	U [Cl$^-$]	U [Ca^{2+}]	U [Mg^{2+}]
Remote vomiting or use of diuretics (> 2 wks)	< 25 mM	< 15 mEq/D	< 10 mM	N: 100–250 mg/d	N to L
Mild K$^+$ deficiency	< 25	< 15	< 10	N	N to L
Severe K$^+$ deficiency	> 25	< 30	> 20	N to H	N to H
HCO$_3^-$ therapy	> 25	> 15	< 10	N	N
Vomiting (current)	> 25	> 15	< 10	N	N to L
Bartter syndrome (current furosemide use)	> 25	> 15	> 20	H to N	N
Gitelman syndrome (current thiazide use)	> 25	> 15	> 20	L < 100 mg/day	H

Abbreviations: H, high; L, low; N, normal.

（三）Treatment of Metabolic Alkalosis

代謝性鹼中毒的治療，最重要的是矯正代謝性鹼中毒的根本病因，此外應注意：

1. 如果在鑑別診斷時發現是「chloride/saline responsive metabolic alkalosis」，代表胞外體液 (extracellular fluid) 容積減少，應給予生理食鹽水 (normal saline) 補充。
2. 如果在鑑別診斷時發現是「chloride unresponsive metabolic alkalosis」，多分成流失性（例如利尿劑、瀉劑、低血鉀、Bartter's, 不會產生新發高血壓）或 renin-angiotensin-aldosterone system 過度活化（會產生新發生／嚴重的高血壓）有關，若是後者可檢驗血中 renin、aldosterone 做進一步鑑別診斷，必要時給予手術或 spironolactone 藥物治療。
3. 合併有低血鉀症者應口服補充鉀離子或者在靜脈輸液中添加適量的氯化鉀，矯正低血鉀才能有效改善代謝性鹼中毒。

延伸閱讀文獻

Berend K, de Vries APJ, Gans ROB. Physiological approach to assessment of acid-base disturbances [published correction appears in *N Engl J Med.* 2014;371(20):1948]. *N Engl J Med.* 2014;371(15):1434-1445. doi:10.1056/NEJMra1003327

Hamm LL, Dubose TD Jr. Disorders of acid-base balance. In: Yu ASL, Chertow GM, Luyckx VA, Marsden PA, Skorecki K, Taal MW, eds. *Brenner and Rector's The Kidney*. 11th ed. Philadelphia, PA: Elsevier; 2020: 496-536.

Chapter 4

Sodium and Potassium

牛志遠
陽明交通大學附設醫院腎臟科

曾偉誠
臺北榮民總醫院腎臟科

鈉和水的平衡，以及它們在不同的身體區間 (body compartments) 的分布，對於體液的恆定 (fluid homeostasis)，特別是血管內的容積非常的重要。全身鈉含量與水分含量改變，會造成血鈉濃度異常，進而對病人的正常生理功能造成嚴重的影響，是臨床上極常見的問題。鉀離子主要的生理功能是維持細胞膜正常的電位差，血鉀濃度異常會造成致命性的心律不整、橫紋肌溶解、癱瘓。如何診斷及處理鉀離子的異常是臨床腎臟學的一項重要技能。鉀離子的異常不只常見於腎臟科的會診，也和血液透析及腎臟移植緊密的相關。

一、學習目標

（一）血鈉濃度異常的鑑別診斷及處置
（二）治療血鈉濃度異常時，血鈉濃度矯正速率限制，及治療速度過快時的可能併發症
（三）血鉀濃度異常的鑑別診斷及處置
（四）低血鉀症及高血鉀症的緊急處理
（五）補充鉀離子的限制及注意事項

二、入門概述

（一）Na$^+$, K$^+$, and Water

1. Na$^+$ 是細胞外最主要的陽離子，K$^+$ 是細胞內最主要的陽離子，細胞內外的離子濃度差以及各離子通道的開關狀態構成膜電位。各離子偏離其平常時的濃度便會改變膜電位，進而造成臨床上看到的諸多症狀。
2. 處理電解質異常前首先要評估全身水分組成。身體水含量約占身體 50%–60% 的體重，因半數的水儲藏於肌肉組織，故肌肉組織（以及無水脂肪組織的多寡）也會影響水在身體內的占比 (Figure 4-1)。

   身體總水量 (total body water, TBW) 的計算：

   $$TBW = BW \times 0.6 \text{ (or 0.5 in woman)}$$

3. 身體內的水約 2/3 在胞內，1/3 在胞外。而在胞外的這 1/3，又會因 plasma albumin 以及微血管內的靜水壓 (hydrostatic pressure) 來改變其在血管內 (25%) 及組織中 (75%) 的比例。

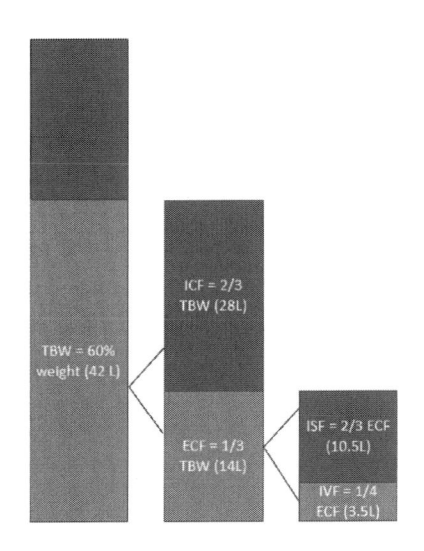

Figure 4-1. 人體不同身體區間 (body compartments) 的水分分布

Abbreviations: ECF, extracellular fluid; ICF, intracellular fluid; ISF, interstitial fluid; IVF, intravascular fluid; TBW, total body water.

4. Na⁺ 和 K⁺ 於人體的分布體積 (volume of distribution) 需以 TBW 計算，而非 extracellular fluid (ECF) 或 intracellular fluid (ICF) 體積，因為若 ECF [Na⁺] 上升，將使水分由 ICF 移至 ECF，直到細胞內外液滲透壓相等。

（二）正常生理對鈉離子濃度的調控

1. 腎小球所過濾的 Na⁺，60% 在近端腎曲小管 (proximal convoluted tubule)，30% 在亨耳氏環上行支 (thick ascending limb of Henle's loop)，7% 在遠端腎曲小管 (distal convoluted tubule)，剩下 2%–3% 在集尿管 (collecting duct, CD) 被再吸收。99% 濾過的鈉都會被回收。
2. 除尿液之外，汗液是低鈉低張（約 30–65 mEq/L），而腸液／膽汁則有較高的鈉離子濃度 (Table 4-1)。
3. 血鈉濃度約等同全身鈉離子量加上全身鉀離子量，再除以 TBW。而身體調控血鈉濃度最快的方式便是透過調控分母，也就是 TBW，主要的機制便是 anti-diuretic hormone (ADH)。

（三）正常生理對水分的調控

1. 正常生理一天尿液最少有 500 mL（600 mOsm 的溶質以最大濃度 1,200 mOsm/kg 的濃縮尿液排出），而呼吸道及皮膚的 insensible loss 約 600 mL（或 8–10 mL/kg of body weight，intubation 及發燒會增加這方面的流失），糞便約 200 mL。

Table 4-1. 不同段的消化道分泌物的電解質濃度 [a]

位置	Na$^+$ (mEq/L)	K$^+$ (mEq/L)	Cl$^-$ (mEq/L)	HCO$_3^-$ (mEq/L)
胃 (stomach)	65	10	100	–
膽汁 (bile)	150	4	100	35
胰臟 (pancreas)	150	7	80	75
十二指腸 (duodenum)	90	15	90	15
中段小腸 (mid-small bowel)	140	6	100	20
末端迴腸 (terminal ileum)	140	8	60	70
直腸 (rectum)	40	90	15	30

[a] 資料參考來源：[1]。

2. 攝取水分不足會增加 ECF 的滲透壓，刺激下視丘引起渴覺，進而分泌 ADH 在 CD 把水分吸收回來，增加尿液的滲透壓。體液容積不足或是 angiotensin-II 也會刺激 ADH，故 effective volume 不足就會持續刺激 ADH 分泌。
3. 諸多因素調控著 ADH 的分泌，故 hypotonicity 時 ADH 並非一定被抑制，要去找其他的 contributing factor。(Nausea is the most prominent non-osmotic stimuli to arginine vasopressin secretion in human.)

（四）正常生理對鉀離子濃度的調控

1. 絕大多數的 K$^+$ 分布在細胞內 (> 98%)，又以肌肉組織占大宗 (75%)。一天的 intake 約 100 mEq，90% 由腎臟排泄，剩下的才由腸胃道排出。在腎功能衰竭的情況下，腸胃排出的比重可到 30%。
2. 腎臟排 K$^+$ 主要在 connecting tubule 和 cortical collecting duct (CCD)。主要的驅力是 epithelial sodium channel (ENaC) 吸收尿腔內的鈉使尿腔轉負電而促使鉀從 Maxi-K 和 renal outer medullary potassium (ROMK) channel 釋放到尿腔中。Aldosterone 可以上調 CCD basolateral membrane 側的 Na$^+$/K$^+$ ATPase 和 apical membrane 側的 ENaC，進而促進留鈉排鉀。

三、低血鈉

（一）起手式

1. 親身評估和密切抽血追蹤最重要
2. 病史詢問

　　Intake 多少，吃了什麼，output 多少，是否有嘔吐或拉肚子，藥物、類固醇、中草藥。

3. 危急程度

(1) Acute or chronic：低血鈉造成症狀的嚴重程度，和低血鈉發生的速度 (acuity of onset) 和低血鈉的程度 (magnitude) 相關。當低血鈉發生時，細胞會吸收水分並腫脹。這樣的情形對於被包覆在顱骨內的大腦會造成嚴重的影響，腦壓會上升。因此腦細胞會藉由排除細胞內的溶質，以減少腦細胞腫脹的程度，這樣的代價大概需要 24–48 小時。考量到腦細胞代價所需的時間，小於 48 小時內發生的低血鈉定義為急性低血鈉 (acute hyponatremia)。發生的速度比濃度的絕對值更為重要。慢性低血鈉因為腦細胞已經發生代價，所以治療需要慢慢來。

(2) 是否已有神經學症狀 (e.g., confusion, ataxia, and seizure)，若有神經學症狀就要積極矯正低血鈉。

(3) 容易產生神經學併發症的危險因子：血鈉 < 105 mEq/L、酗酒、肝硬化、營養不良及低血鉀。

4. 是不是真的低血鈉

(1) Hypertonic（假的）：effective osmole 把水拉到血管內稀釋電解質濃度。例如：mannitol、glucose（每 100 mg/dL 的上升降低 [Na^+] 1.6–2.4 mEq/L）。在糖尿病酮症酸中毒 (diabetic ketoacidosis) 及高血糖高滲透壓狀態 (hyperglycemic hyperosmolar state) 時，此原則非常重要。

(2) Isotonic（假的）：現已少見。血中的 protein、lipid 太多造成血清所占比例下降，此時若以間接離子選擇性電極法 (indirect ion-selective electrode) 來測定血鈉濃度會出現假性偏低。

5. Check List

(1) Serum: osmolality, Na^+, K^+, Cl^-, blood urea nitrogen (BUN), creatinine (Cr), Glu, Chol, TG, total protein, uric acid.（懷疑 syndrome of inappropriate antidiuretic hormone secretion [SIADH] 時）

(2) Urine: U_{Osm} (osmolality), U_{Na}, U_{Cr}, U_{UA}, U_{Cl}

（二）開始 Differential Diagnosis (D/D)

1. 低血鈉病人的鑑別診斷

診斷低血鈉的流程圖請參考 Figure 4-2

2. U_{Osm} 的評估（ADH 是否正確被抑制以排出最稀釋的尿液？）

U_{Osm} < 100 mOsm/kg：ADH 有正確被抑制，但是怎麼還是水比鈉多？

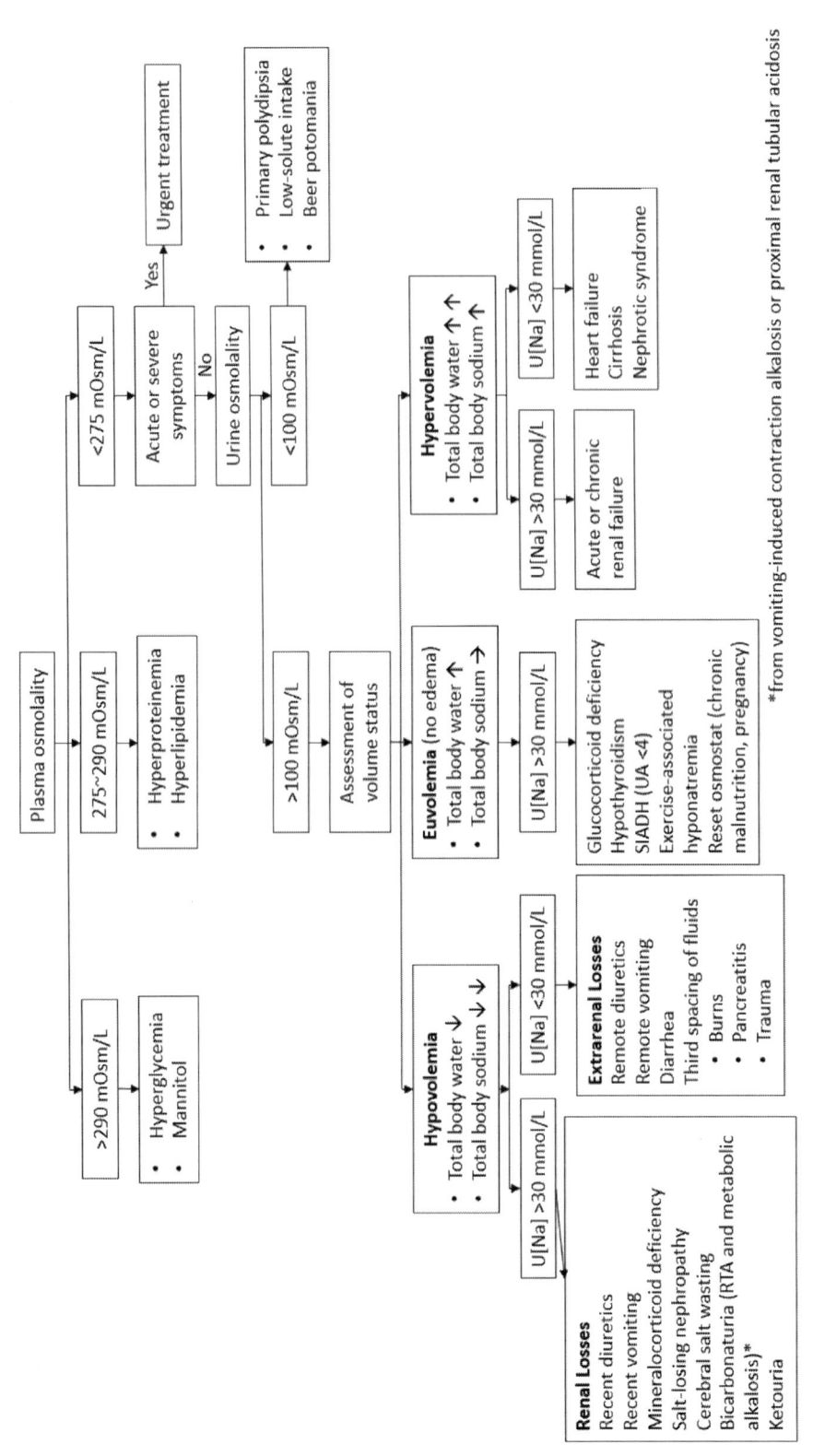

Figure 4-2. 低血鈉病人的鑑別診斷

Plasma osmolality

- **>290 mOsm/L**
  - Hyperglycemia
  - Mannitol

- **275~290 mOsm/L**
  - Hyperproteinemia
  - Hyperlipidemia

- **<275 mOsm/L**
  - Acute or severe symptoms
    - Yes → Urgent treatment
    - No → Urine osmolality
      - <100 mOsm/L
        - Primary polydipsia
        - Low-solute intake
        - Beer potomania
      - >100 mOsm/L → Assessment of volume status

Hypovolemia
- Total body water ↓
- Total body sodium ↓↓

  - U[Na] <30 mmol/L → **Extrarenal Losses**
    - Remote diuretics
    - Remote vomiting
    - Diarrhea
    - Third spacing of fluids
      - Burns
      - Pancreatitis
      - Trauma

  - U[Na] >30 mmol/L → **Renal Losses**
    - Recent diuretics
    - Recent vomiting
    - Mineralocorticoid deficiency
    - Salt-losing nephropathy
    - Cerebral salt wasting
    - Bicarbonaturia (RTA and metabolic alkalosis)*
    - Ketouria

Euvolemia (no edema)
- Total body water ↑
- Total body sodium →

  - U[Na] >30 mmol/L
    - Glucocorticoid deficiency
    - Hypothyroidism
    - SIADH (UA <4)
    - Exercise-associated hyponatremia
    - Reset osmostat (chronic malnutrition, pregnancy)

Hypervolemia
- Total body water ↑↑
- Total body sodium ↑

  - U[Na] >30 mmol/L
    - Acute or chronic renal failure

  - U[Na] <30 mmol/L
    - Heart failure
    - Cirrhosis
    - Nephrotic syndrome

*from vomiting-induced contraction alkalosis or proximal renal tubular acidosis

Abbreviations: RTA, renal tubular acidosis; SIADH, syndrome of inappropriate antidiuretic hormone secretion.

(1) Low-solute intake 或 polydipsia：假設一天只吃 120 mOsm 的溶質，那最稀的尿液濃度也只有 60 mOsm/kg，於是一天為了排這 120 mOsm 只能夠排 2 L 的水，喝超過 2 L 的都會變成 free water retention，因此造成低血鈉。

(2) U_{Osm} < 100 mOsm/kg，可以幫助診斷 primary polydipsia, low-solute intake (tea and toast syndrome, beer potomania)。

(3) U_{Osm} 越高時，越像是 SIADH。

(4) U_{Osm} 對治療低血鈉時的溶液選擇非常重要。

3. 進行體液狀態的評估

(1) 病史、理學檢查 (physical examination) 和輔助的實驗室檢查。病人是否有噁心、嘔吐、拉肚子、大量流汗？diabetes mellitus (DM) poor control？尿量如何？是否有管路 (drain)？藥物像是 thiazide、desmopressin (DDAVP)、non-steroidal anti-inflammatory drug (NSAID)？pancreatitis？

(2) Hypovolemic，水少但鈉更少，乾巴巴的臨床上通常最好判斷：
   A. 額外輔助的 lab：Serum BUN/Cr > 20, U_{Na} < 30 mEq/L（身體覺得 volume 不夠瘋狂吸鈉），U_{Osm} > 500 mOsm/kg, serum albumin、hematocrit 不合理的高（濃縮效應）。
   B. 利用 U_{Na} (30 mEq/L) 區分是 renal loss 還是 extra-renal loss。若要使用 fractional excretion of sodium (FENa) (1%) 來鑑別，baseline 的腎功能必須是正常的。

(3) Isovolemic，水不正常滯留，但鈉總量還好故 ECF 沒有到 hypervolemic
   A. Stress 是最常見造成 SIADH 的原因，其他常見的原因請參考 Table 4-2。要記得排除 hypothyroidism 和 adrenal insufficiency。
   B. SIADH 的診斷標準 (diagnostic criteria) 及 SIADH 常見的臨床表徵如 Table 4-3。U_{Na} > 30 mEq/L 代表身體並非 ECF 不夠而留鈉而是單純 ADH 過多。

(4) Hypervolemic，鈉多水更多，要找背後的 systemic 原因才能治本。
   A. Effective volume 不足，活化 renin-angiotensin-aldosterone system (RAAS) 和刺激 ADH 生成，造成 U_{Na} < 10 mEq/L，FENa < 1%，例如 congestive heart failure (CHF)、cirrhosis、nephrotic syndrome 等。
   B. Excessive Na^+ load 或是水相較於鈉排不出去，像是 renal failure。

（三）開始治療

1. 快速地使血鈉上升，是用增加併發症的風險來減少住院天數。在無明顯症狀的病人上不值得。低血鈉治療目標不僅只是 correct lab value 而是找出潛在病因以避免再次發生。

Table 4-2. Syndrome of inappropriate antidiuresis hormone secretion 的常見原因 [a]

惡性腫瘤	肺部疾病	中樞神經系統疾病	藥物	其他
上皮細胞癌	感染	感染	刺激抗利尿激素分泌或增加強其效果的藥物	遺傳性抗利尿激素 V2 受體的功能獲得型突變 (gain-of-function mutations)
肺部	細菌性肺炎	腦炎	Chlorpropamide	原發性 (idiopathic)
小細胞肺癌	病毒性肺炎	腦膜炎	SSRIs	暫時性的
間皮瘤	肺膿瘍	腦膿瘍	Tricyclic antidepressants	耐力運動
口咽	結核病	落磯山斑疹熱	Clofibrate	全身麻醉
腸胃道腫瘤	麴菌病	人類免疫缺乏病毒感染	Carbamazepine	噁心
胃		出血及腫塊	Vincristine	痛
十二指腸		硬腦膜下血腫	Nicotine	壓力
胰臟	囊腫性纖維化	蜘蛛膜下腔出血	Narcotics	
	呼吸衰竭且接受正壓呼吸	腦中風	Antipsychotic drugs	
泌尿生殖系統		腦腫瘤	Ifosfamide	
輸尿管		頭部外傷	Cyclophosphamide	
膀胱		水腦症	NSAIDs	
前列腺癌		海綿竇血栓	MDMA (ecstasy)	
子宮內膜		其他	抗利尿激素的類似物	
胸腺腫瘤		多發性硬化症	DDAVP	
淋巴瘤		Guillain-Barré 症候群	Oxytocin	
惡性肉瘤		Shy-Drager 症候群	Vasopressin	
尤文氏肉瘤 (Ewing's sarcoma)		震顫性譫妄 (delirium tremens)		
		急性衛歇性紫質症		

Abbreviations: DDAVP, desmopressin; MDMA, 3,4-Methylenedioxymethamphetamine; NSAID, non-steroidal anti-inflammatory drug; SSRIs, selective serotonin reuptake inhibitors.

[a] 資料參考來源：[2]。

Table 4-3. SIADH 的診斷標準 (diagnostic criteria) 及 SIADH 常見的臨床表徵

SIADH 常見的臨床表徵
Bartter & Schwartz 的 SIADH 診斷標準
• 低滲透壓低血鈉 (effective S_{Osm} < 275 mOsm/kg H_2O)。
• 等容積狀態 (euvolemia)。
• 小便沒有被最大幅度的稀釋 (U_{Osm} > 100 mOsm/kg H_2O)。
• 在正常的鹽分和水分攝取的情況下，有上升的尿鈉排除量，且沒有鹽分滯留的情形 (U_{Na} > 30 mEq/L)。
• 沒有肝硬化、心臟衰竭或嚴重的慢性腎臟病。
• 沒有其他等容積低滲透壓低血鈉的替代診斷，像是甲狀腺機能低下症、腎上腺機能不全或是利尿劑的使用。
其他支持診斷 SIADH 的資訊
• 尿酸 < 4 mg/dL。
• 尿酸排出率 > 10%–12%。
• 給予患者靜脈輸注生理食鹽水後，反而造成血鈉下降。
• 血液中抗利尿激素或和肽素 (copeptin) 的濃度相對於血液的滲透壓有不適當的上升。
• 對於水負荷測試有異常的反應（當給予患者每 kg 體重 20 mL 的水分，於 4 個小時後，水分的排出量小於給予量的 80% 且小便無法被稀釋到滲透壓小於 100 mOsm/kg H_2O）。

Abbreviation: SIADH, syndrome of inappropriate antidiuretic hormone secretion.

2. [Na^+] 上升的速率 < 0.3–0.5 mEq/L/hr，一天的上升量 < 8 mEq/L/day。血鈉濃度上升過快可以用 DDAVP (2 g Q6H) 或 free water rescue (D5W、D10W)。請一定小心不要快速矯正，因為：

(1) 胞外鈉濃度上升過快會讓胞內的水快速跑出來造成 cell shrinkage，myelin sheath 就拉斷了 → 造成 osmotic demyelination syndrome (ODS)，幾天後出現典型的 paraplegia、dysarthria 與 dysphagia，不可逆。

(2) 在補充鈉時，建議可以使用 Adrogué 等人 [3] 評估每公升的高鈉溶液會讓血鈉上升多少。

$$TBW = \text{lean body weight (in kilograms)} \times 0.6 \text{（男性）or} \times 0.5 \text{（女性）}$$

這個公式假定沒有正在流失的電解質或水分，因此只是粗略的估計。

$$\text{Change in serum } Na^+ = \frac{(\text{infusate } Na^+ + \text{infusate } K^+) - \text{serum } Na^+}{\text{total body water} + 1}$$

(3) 治療過程中，應頻繁追蹤血鈉濃度（可考慮至少每 6 小時一次），避免矯正過快。

3. 在 Hypervolemic：採限水，並同時使用 furosemide 讓身體排出過多水分，或是改善 effective volume 不足 (CHF and cirrhosis) 來去除刺激 ADH 分泌的情況（最困難）。
4. Isovolemic：限水，也可使用 furosemide 增加排水來降低 urine osmolality，可增加鹽分、蛋白質攝取（增加溶質 → osmotic diuresis）。
5. Hypovolemic：half 至 normal saline (NS) 慢慢滴慢慢矯正，要切記改善 effective volume 不足的時候就會讓 ADH 分泌下降 → 尿液變稀排水變多 → 血鈉上升更快。
6. Urine osmolality 的重要性：

假設 U_{Osm} = 600 mOsm/kg，intravenous (IV) 給予 1 L 的 NS，裡面有約 150 mEq 的 Na^+ 和 150 mEq 的 Cl^-，一共 300 mEq 的溶質在 1 L 的水中。為了排這 300 mEq 的溶質，U_{Osm} = 600 的病人只需 0.5 L 的尿液，於是增加了 0.5 L 的 free water，血鈉更低。

（四）為什麼低血鉀是治療低血鈉症產生神經學症狀之 Risk Factor？為何補鉀就可補鈉？

1. 鉀為胞內主要 osmole，鉀不足細胞就會更容易 shrinkage → 加重 ODS 的機轉。
2. 當我們補充鉀離子時，這些多的鉀為了維持一定的胞外血鉀濃度便會跑去胞內，並交換胞內的鈉出來以維持電中性。此外，胞內的鉀越多也會吸引更多的水進入胞內，降低 ECF，血鈉濃度便因此上升了。
3. 因此實務上我們可以把鉀視同鈉來補充，甚至更好用，只要

$$([Na^+] + [K^+])_{Infusate} - ([Na^+] + [K^+])_{Serum} > 20 \ mEq/L$$

就可以補充，例如用 0.45% saline (77 mEq/L) 500 mL + 15% KCl 15 mL (60 mEq/L) = 137 mEq/L

四、高血鈉

（一）起手式

高血鈉 = 身體的水比鈉少，為什麼水留不住或無法取得？找水從哪裡流失，然後節流 + 開源。

（二）開始 D/D

1. 診斷高血鈉的流程圖請參考 Figure 4-3。

Hypernatremia

Urine osmolality

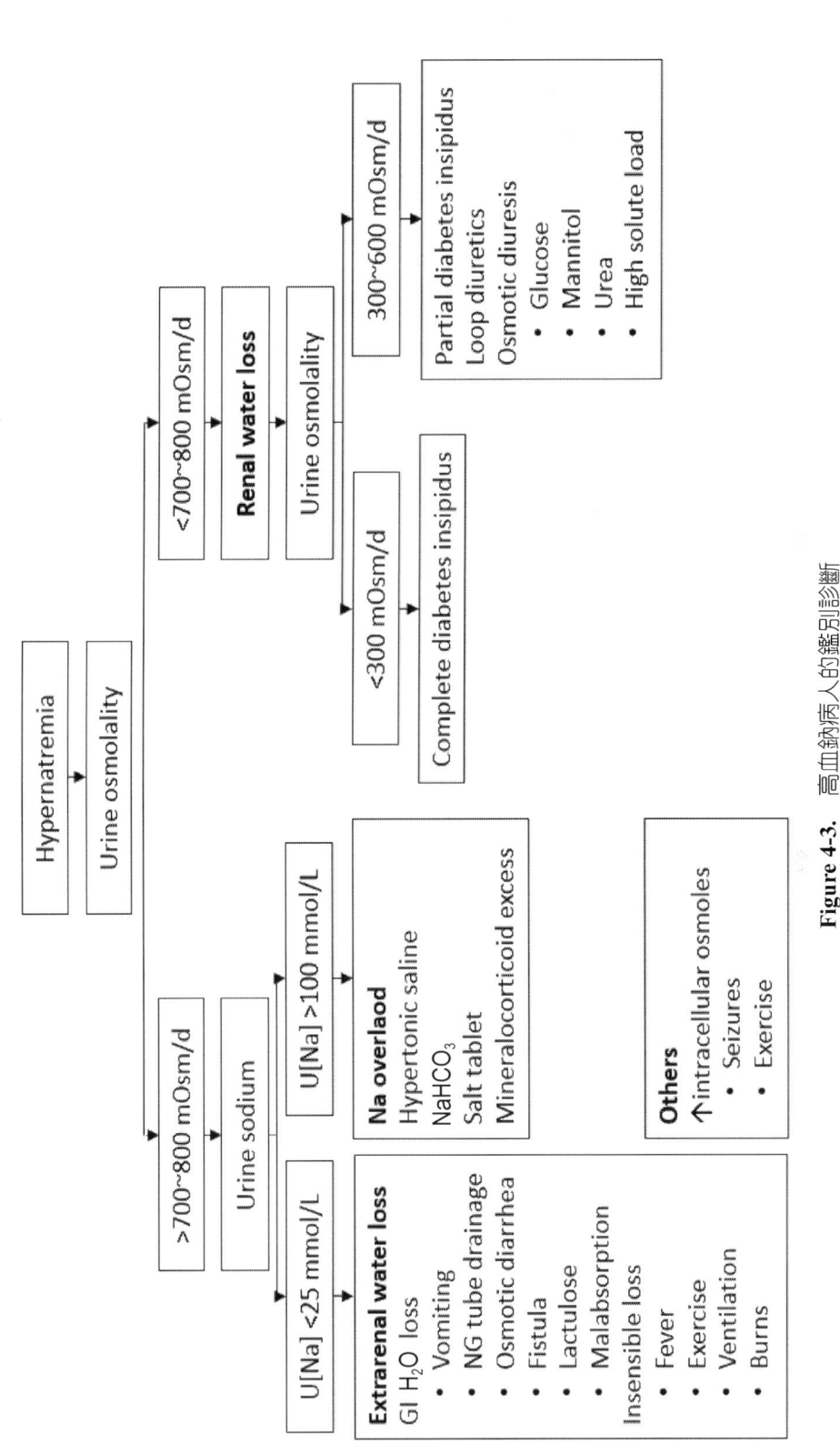

- **>700~800 mOsm/d** → Urine sodium
  - **U[Na] <25 mmol/L**
    - **Extrarenal water loss**
      GI H₂O loss
      - Vomiting
      - NG tube drainage
      - Osmotic diarrhea
      - Fistula
      - Lactulose
      - Malabsorption

      Insensible loss
      - Fever
      - Exercise
      - Ventilation
      - Burns
  - **U[Na] >100 mmol/L**
    - **Na overload**
      - Hypertonic saline
      - NaHCO₃
      - Salt tablet
      - Mineralocorticoid excess
    - **Others**
      ↑intracellular osmoles
      - Seizures
      - Exercise

- **<700~800 mOsm/d** → **Renal water loss** → Urine osmolality
  - **<300 mOsm/d**
    - Complete diabetes insipidus
  - **300~600 mOsm/d**
    - Partial diabetes insipidus
    - Loop diuretics
    - Osmotic diuresis
      - Glucose
      - Mannitol
      - Urea
      - High solute load

Figure 4-3. 高血鈉病人的鑑別診斷

Abbreviation: GI, gastrointestinal tract; NG tube, nasogastric tube.

2. 高血鈉一定是 hyperosmolality，所以直接從理應被大量分泌的 ADH 著手。
3. U_{Osm} > 700–800 mOsm/kg

   ADH 正常分泌與作用，暗示水分流失並非腎源性，以 GI (gastrointestinal, GI) tract 與 insensible loss 最常見，燒燙傷患者也屬此類。少數是外來的 sodium load 太大，請 survey intravenous fluid (IVF) 和 medication。
4. U_{Osm} < 700–800 mOsm/kg

   (1) Diuresis due to osmotic agents (urea, glucose, and mannitol) 或 diuretics，尿中有大量溶質順便帶走更大量的水，故 U_{Osm} 落在中間。

   (2) 尿崩症 (diabetes insipidus)，因 ADH 不足 (central) 或 resistance (nephrogenic)。

   (3) Central diabetes insipitus (DI) 通常可以由病史推測（產後女性尤其注意 Sheehan syndrome）。ADH 在下視丘中製造，posterior pituitary 儲存及分泌。若僅破壞 posterior pituitary，則 ADH 製造正常，分泌可改到 median eminence 的血管網中釋放，故 pituitary adenoma 造成 Central DI 並不常見，要想到其他診斷。

   　　A. Craniopharyngioma（會引起 median eminence 的傷害）。

   　　B. Rapid enlarging sellar or suprasellar masses.

   　　C. Granulomatous disease with more diffuse hypothalamic involvement.

   (4) Nephrogenic DI 更為常見，且多為後天

   　　A. Drugs: lithium（精神科）, foscarnet, cidofovir, and demeclocycline.

   　　B. 電解質問題：hypercalcemia、hypokalemia。

   　　C. 病史：post-obstructive diuresis, recovery phase of acute tubular necrosis, polycystic kidney disease, Sjogren's syndrome, amyloidosis, pregnancy（胎盤製造的 cysteine aminopeptidase [= vasopressinase] 在血中分解 ADH）。

   　　D. Central 和 Nephrogenic DI 的確診和區分傳統上是透過 water deprivation test（限水試驗）和施打 DDAVP。限水試驗可能會造成電解質急性或劇烈變動，會產生危險，請務必跟總醫師和主治醫師討論。

（三）開始治療

1. 再次提醒，身體的奧祕總有意外，密切的追蹤不可取代，治療過程中，應頻繁追蹤血鈉濃度（可考慮每 6 小時一次），避免矯正過快。
2. 高血鈉矯正過快，胞外鈉離子快速降低會讓水分讓相對高鈉的細胞內移動，造成 brain edema，雖然沒有 ODS 那麼絕望，但一樣要小心。

   在補充 free water 時，也可以使用 Adrogué 等人 [3]，評估每公升的低鈉溶液會讓血鈉下降多少。須注意因為高血鈉是水分限縮的情況，此時 TBW = lean body weight (in kilograms) × 0.5（男性）or × 0.4（女性）。

$$\text{Change in serum Na}^+ = \frac{(\text{infusate Na}^+ + \text{infusate K}^+) - \text{serum Na}^+}{\text{total body water} + 1}$$

3. Osmotic diuresis 的治療就是減少尿中的 osmotic agent。
4. Nephrogenic diabetes insipidus (DI) 請 correct underlying disease，並可利用 Thiazide 減少 ECF 的方式來增加 ADH 分泌。Pregnancy 的 vasopressinase 可使用 DDAVP 來克服（DDAVP 是 V2 agonist 較不易被分解）。Lithium 造成的 nephrogenic DI 可使用 Amiloride 來改善。且因後天性 nephrogenic DI 對 ADH 常只有部分阻抗性，若上述治療方式無效，也可考慮加上 DDAVP。
5. Central DI 可以使用 DDAVP，但請一定用超低劑量開始並且追蹤血鈉。

五、低血鉀

（一）起手式

1. 是真、假（Pseudohypokalemia as in 血中白血球 > 10^6/μL）還是 Transcellular Shift？

　　Alkalosis、insulin、hypokalemic periodic paralysis、acute increase in cell production (megaloblastic anemia under treatment with B12, acute myeloid leukemia crisis)、hypothermia、high adrenergic states（e.g., 氣喘或 chronic obstructive pulmonary disease 發作、急性心肌梗塞、頭部受傷、服用大量咖啡因、安非他命類藥物、theophylline、$β_2$ agonist 等）、鋇劑中毒或 chloroquine 過量（關閉細胞膜 K^+ channel）。

2. 低血鉀的症狀以及後遺症

　　Electrocardiography changes: U wave, broad flat T waves, ST depression, QT prolongation（尤其 hypoK 常合併 hypoMg，又一個 long QT 的 risk factor）(Table 4-4)。

（二）開始 D/D

1. 首先評估 K^+ 從哪裡流失。推薦使用 Spot urine K^+/Cr ratio（不用留 24 小時小便，可即時透過單次尿液評估）。若 ratio 大於 2.0 mmol/mmol 或 15 mmol/g 則表示 renal loss (high K^+ excretion)。（注意上下的單位，若選擇 mmol/g，本院 Urine K^+ 的單位是 mmol/L，而 Urine Cr 的單位是 mg/dL，所以相除之比值要再乘以 100 才是 mmol/g）。
    (1) Transtubular potassium gradient (TTKG) 公式的來由：TTKG 代表的是 K^+ 分泌到 CCD 的能力。故要比較的就是在 CCD 時的尿腔鉀濃度和 peritubular capillary 之血鉀濃度，尿 K_{CCD}／血 K_{CCD} 比值越大代表分泌能力越強。

Table 4-4. 低血鉀的臨床症狀與表徵[a]

項目	臨床症狀與表徵
心臟	心律不整、心肌收縮力下降、血壓上升、增加毛地黃類藥物毒性。
腎臟	在慢性低血鉀狀況下，腎絲球濾過率及腎血流下降、腎臟濃縮小便能力下降導致多尿、腎臟對鈉、檸檬酸及重碳酸根重吸收增加導致高血壓、低檸檬酸尿症及代謝性鹼中毒、腎囊泡形成，甚至導致慢性腎臟病。
肌肉	腸胃道蠕動減少、膀胱收縮力減少導致膀胱擴大、橫紋肌溶解、肌肉無力癱瘓。
周邊神經	感覺異常、肌腱反射減少。
新陳代謝	（慢性低血鉀狀況下）醛固酮（aldosterone）分泌減少、增加胰島素抗性、增加腎素（renin）分泌、增加腎臟產氨作用（ammoniagenesis）。

[a] 資料參考來源：[4]。

    (2) 但 CCD 尿腔內的鉀濃度是多少呢？只能從自膀胱所排出的 urine [K⁺] 來回推，所以我們假設 CCD 之後只有水分吸收，而沒有鉀的吸收分泌（故 TTKG 假設 ADH 有作用）。

    (3) 正常情況下 CCD 為 iso-osmolar zone，所以可用 serum Osm 來代表在 CCD 的 urine OsmCCD，再和最後排出的 urine Osm^{urine} 來比較，我們就知道這段過程中尿液濃縮了多少倍，也就可以推知在濃縮前，CCD 內的尿 K$_{CCD}$ 究竟是多少。

$$TTKG = \frac{[K^+]_{CCD}}{[K^+]_{serum}} = \frac{[K^+]_{urine} \times \left(Osm_{serum}/Osm_{urine}\right)}{[K^+]_{serum}} = \frac{[K^+]_{urine}/Osm_{urine}}{[K^+]_{serum}/Osm_{serum}}$$

    (4) TTKG 僅適用於 U_{Na}^+ > 25 mEq/L，且 urine Osm ≥ serum Osm。

2. Urine K⁺/Cr < 15 mmol/g，歸在 low renal K⁺ excretion，多數是因為 GI loss 或是 transcellular shift，少數是因長期鉀離子 intake 不足。這其中還可以藉由酸鹼狀態進一步區分可能的成因。

    (1) GI 流失 HCO$_3^-$ 和 K⁺，故呈現 metabolic acidosis 以及腎臟留鉀，造成 U_K/U_{Cr} 低。

    (2) Remote diuretics 因 volume contraction 而造成 metabolic alkalosis。

    (3) Vomiting, NG (nasogastric) drainage 因為流失的是 HCl 故呈現的往往是 metabolic alkalosis，而引發的 bicarbonaturia 加上 secondary hyperaldosteronism 造成 Urine K⁺ 排泄增加。

3. Urine K⁺/Cr > 15 mmol/g，則屬 high renal K⁺ excretion，此時要先評估病人臨床上是否有 mineralocorticoid excess 的證據，所以我們接著從血壓和 fluid/volume status 來評估 RAAS 相關路徑是否被活化 (Figure 4-4)。

Hypokalemia due to renal loss with hypertension or elevated volume status

- Renin ↑ Aldosterone ↑
  - Renal artery stenosis
  - Renin-secreting tumor
  - Malignant hypertension
  - Pheochromocytoma

- Renin ↓ Aldosterone ↑
  - Primary aldosteronism
    - Bilateral adrenal hyperplasia
    - Adrenal adenoma
    - Glucocorticoid-remediable aldosteronism

- Renin ↓ Aldosterone ↓
  - Cortisol ↓
    - Congenital adrenal hyperplasia
      - 11β-hydroxylase deficiency
      - 17α-hydroxylase deficiency
  - Cortisol →
    - Apparent mineralocorticoid excess*
    - Licorice ingestion
    - Carbenoxolone ingestion
    - Aldosterone analogue (Fludrocortisone)
    - Deoxycorticosterone producing tumor
    - Liddle's syndrome
  - Cortisol ↑
    - Cushing's syndrome
    - Ectopic ACTH syndrome
    - Exogenous glucocorticoids

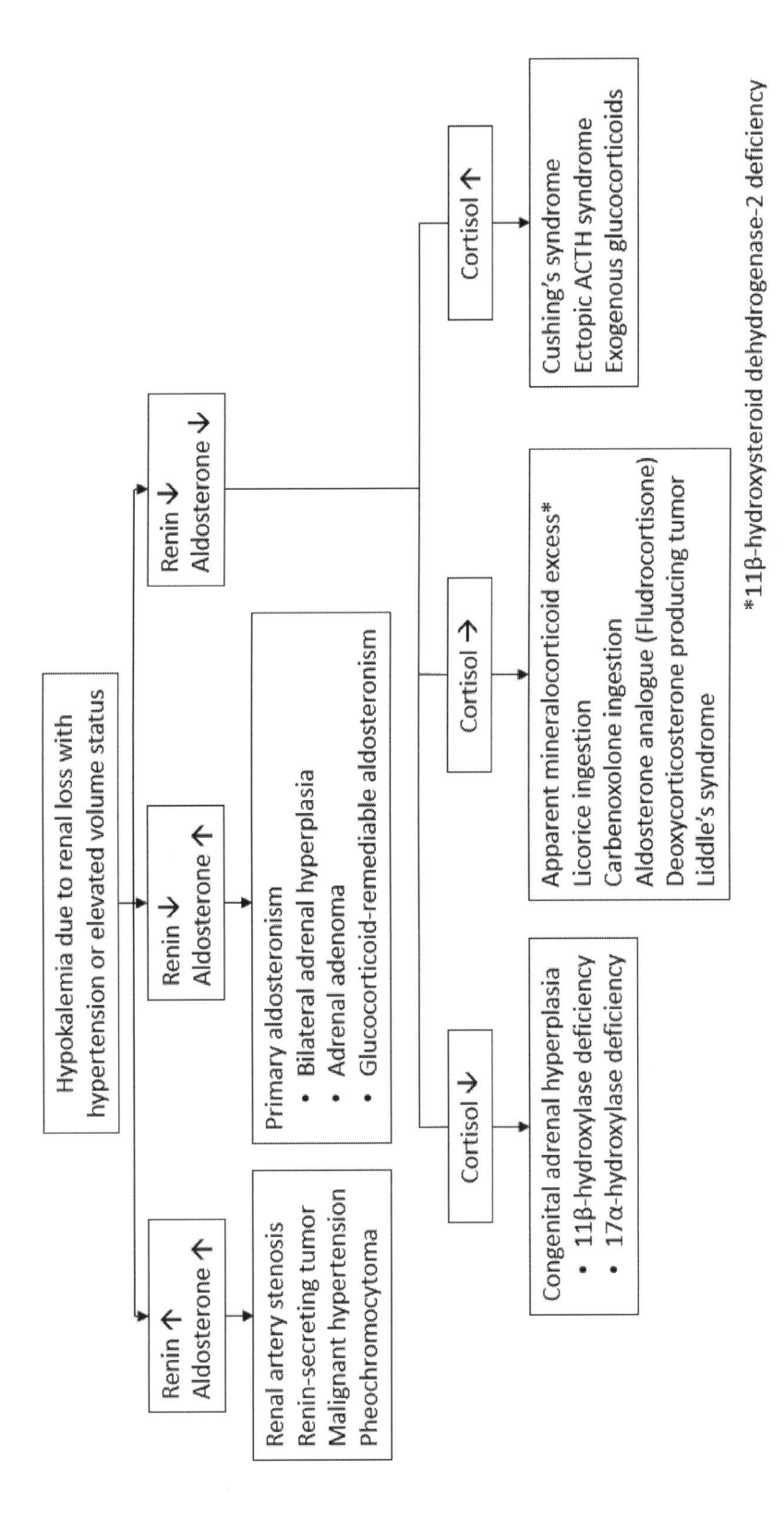

*11β-hydroxysteroid dehydrogenase-2 deficiency

Figure 4-4. 低血鉀同時合併高血壓或是體液容積過多時的鑑別診斷

Abbreviation: ACTH, adrenocorticotropic hormone.

(1) RAAS 最上游的 renin 就開始高了，下游的 aldosterone 也因而升高，有 renin-secreting tumor、RVH (renal vascular hypertension) 等（Figure 4-4 最左邊）。

(2) 中游的 aldosterone 過多，renin 被回饋抑制而低的則有原發性醛固酮症 (primary aldosteronism) 的病人（Figure 4-4 中間）。

(3) 最下游的，像是 Liddle's syndrome、apparent mineralocorticoid excess、服用 licorice、cortisol 過多或 cortisol 製造過程中的 11-deoxycorticosterone (DOC) 過度累積 (congenital adrenal hyperplasia, 11β-hydroxylase 或 17α-hydroxylase deficiency)（Figure 4-4 最右邊）。

4. 血壓和 fluid/volume status 沒有顯著增加的病人，接著用酸鹼來區分是否為 renal tubular acidosis (RTA) 相關。

   (1) 用 urine NH_4^+ 來看腎臟是否能正常排酸，計算的方式是 urine osmolal gap (UOG) 的一半 UOG= Urine osmolality (Meaured)-Urine osmolality (Calculated) = 2 × Urine NH_4^+（過往用 urine anion gap 來推估代謝性酸中毒時腎臟排出 NH_4^+ 能力的方式，特定狀態下會受到過量未知陰離子的干擾，像是大量的 bicarbonate, penicillin, ketoacid 和 hippurate [toluene 的代謝物，glue-sniffer] 等）

   (2) Cutoff 則是抓在 Urine NH_4^+/U_{Cr} = 3 mmol/mmol，以下算 low → 包含 RTA 以及會引起類似 distal RTA 表徵的 amphotericin B (H^+ back diffusion)。

   (3) 特殊藥物相關

      A. Non-reabsorbable anions 造成尿腔負電性上升，像是 penicillin、nafcillin、dicloxacillin、ticarcillin、oxacillin、carbenicillin。

      B. K^+ 和 Mg^{2+} wasting：amphotericin、foscarnet、cisplatin、ifosfamide、cetuximab。

5. Metabolic alkalosis 的部分比較單純。惟因 alkalosis 的時候，過量而被濾出的 HCO_3^- 會和一部分的 Na^+ 結合故增加 Na^+ 的排泄量。因此我們改以 Urine Cl^- 來評估。

   (1) Urine Cl^- 減少 (< 10 mEq/L)，就是吐胃酸 (HCl) 和 Cl^--losing diarrhea

   (2) Urine Cl^- 增加 (> 20 mEq/L)，則利用尿鈣是否增加來區分 Bartter syndrome (furosemide) 和 Gitelman syndrome (thiazide)。

6. 最後再來看一下低血鉀的流程圖 (Figure 4-5)

（三）開始治療

1. 要補多少？

(1) 無症狀 < 3 mEq/L 還是補。

(2) 心律不整高危險病人要補到 4.0–4.5 mEq/L (acute myocardial infarction, arrhythmia, heart failure, ischemic heart, and under digoxin)，此外肝不好及高血壓也建議血鉀補到 4 mEq/L 以上。

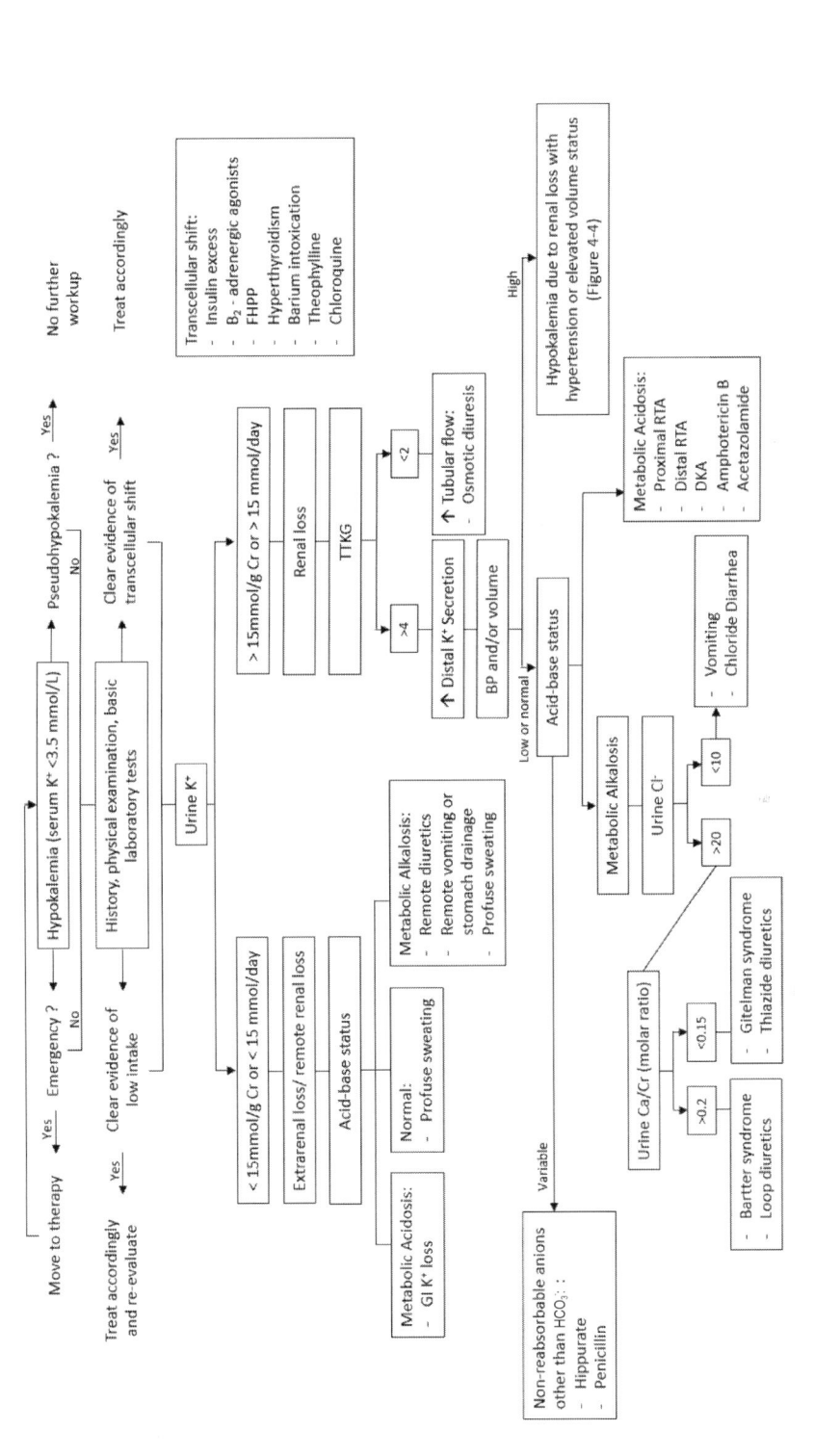

Figure 4-5. 高血鉀鑑別診斷 [a]

Abbreviations: BP, blood pressure; CCD, cortical collecting duct; DKA, diabetic ketoacidosis; FHPP, familial hypokalemic periodic paralysis; GI, gastrointestinal; RTA, renal tubular acidosis; TTKG, transtubular potassium gradient.

[a] 資料參考來源：[4,5]。

Chapter 4 Sodium and Potassium

2. 從哪裡補？

不管是途徑的選擇或是劑量的分配，口服都優先於靜脈補充。如果聽不見腸音，口服補充則不可行。靜脈補充的限制如 Table 4-5。

3. 製劑選擇

(1) 低血鉀合併 alkalosis 時建議使用 KCl 或 K gluconate。
(2) 低血鉀合併 acidosis 時可用碳酸氫鉀（$KHCO_3$，本院無）或檸檬酸鉀（potassium citrate，本院是 U-citra，一包約 30 mEq 的 K^+）或 Potassium gluconate。
(3) 低血鉀合併營養不良時可用磷酸鉀（potassium phosphate, K_3PO_4），此藥含鉀量極高，補充時請務必小心，緩慢給予。
(4) 或以高鉀的食物作補充。

4. 如何減少鉀離子流失

(1) ↓ dose of non-K sparing diuretics
(2) 使用 K^+ sparing medications (e.g., ACEi, ARB, K^+ sparing diuretics, β-blockers)
(3) ↓ Na^+ intake
(4) Hypokalemia due to UGI loss (NG loss, vomiting) → 用 proton pump inhibitor 減少 secretion

5. 特殊注意事項

(1) Thyrotoxicosis、hypokalemic periodic paralyses 的病人以 non-selective β-blocker 為治療主軸，鉀離子補充為輔助，因為可能發生 rebound hyperkalemia。
(2) 低血鎂會導致頑固性的低血鉀與心律不整，因此同時補充鎂離子可以幫助血鉀濃度的提升與避免心律不整的發生。

Table 4-5. 靜脈補充血鉀的濃度及流速限制

	週邊靜脈給予	中心靜脈給予	需心電圖監視器
$[K^+]$ 濃度 輸注速率	≤ 40 mmol/L 輕微低血鉀： ≤ 10 mmol/hr 嚴重低血鉀： ≤ 20 mmol/hr	≤ 100 mmol/L ≤ 20 mmol/hr 當輸注速率超過 20 mmol/hr，需要心電圖監視器	> 60 mmol/L 當血鉀小於 3 mmol/L、病人有心律不整之風險或是低鉀相關的嚴重症狀時： > 20 mmol/hr or > 10 mmol/hr

六、高血鉀

（一）起手式

高血鉀的原因幾乎都可以從低血鉀的機制反過來推，但是治療上則是 medical emergency。

（二）開始 D/D

1. 一樣先排除 Pseudohyperkalemia

IVF with K^+, hemolysis during venipuncture, thrombocytosis, or leukocytosis.

2. 區分 Transcellular Shift

Acidemia, insulin deficiency (DM), β-blockers, digoxin toxicity, massive cellular necrosis, (tumor lysis, rhabdomyolysis, ischemic bowel, and hemolysis), hyperkalemic periodic paralysis、succinylcholine.（機制：K^+ efflux through AChRs-associated cation channels）

3. 接著要評估的是腎臟排出 K^+ 的能力

(1) Distal Na^+ delivery 不夠？（ENaC 吸收鈉是 ROMK 排出鉀的原動力）
   這裡抓的閾值 Urinary Na^+ < 25 mmol/L。
(2) Urinary flow 不夠？（Maxi-K/BK channel 負責 flow-dependent K^+ secretion）
   A. tubule 分泌鉀離子能力正常 (TTKG > 8)，但是 K^+ 總分泌的量不夠(U_K < 40 mmol/day)。
   B. 原因：ECF 不足或是 advanced kidney failure（estimated Glomerular filtration rate < 20 mL/min，尿很少）。
(3) Aldosterone 不夠或是作用不好？
   我們使用 α-fludrocortisone（本院：Florinef）來做鑑別診斷。

4. 給 α-Fludrocortisone 後 TTKG 有改善 (> 8)

代表本來是 aldosterone 製造不足的狀況，那我們要接下來看 aldosterone 的上游 renin 分泌的情況：
(1) 高 renin：先天或後天 primary hypoaldosteronism。
(2) 低 renin：先天或後天 secondary hypoaldosteronism。

A. 常見後天因素：DM、old age、renal insufficiency、systemic lupus erythematosus (SLE)、multiple myeloma、acute glomerulonephritis。

B. Interstitial nephritis 減少 renin 分泌。

C. 藥物：NSAID、COX-2 inhibitor、aliskiren、β-blocker。

5. 若給了 α-fludrocortisone 後 TTKG 卻沒改善 (< 8)

則代表是 renal tubules 對 aldosterone 產生了阻抗性。

(1) Hyperkalemic distal RTA：SLE, sickle cell anemia, and amyloidosis.

(2) Pseudohypoaldosteronism-I.

(3) Calcineurin inhibitors (cyclosporine, tacrolimus).

（二）開始治療

1. 依照時間順序，先處理最可能致命的狀況，然後快速把胞外的鉀移入胞內，然後再減少攝取，增加排除，真正減少身體裡的鉀。

2. 用鈣拮抗高血鉀的 cardiac arrhythmogenic effect

    (1) 機制：action potential threshold ↑, excitability ↓.

    (2) Effect starts in 1–3 mins, lasts for 30–60 mins.

    (3) Calcium gluconate, drug of choice.

    (4) Calcium chloride，extravasation 會造成 tissue necrosis，故建議可用 central line，否則需小心靜脈注射給藥。

3. 把 K^+ 從胞外趕到細胞內（最快降鉀的方式）

    (1) Insulin and glucose：首選

        A. Infusion: RI 10 U in D10W 500 mL, IVD for 60 mins.

        B. Bolus: RI 10 U IVA followed by D50W 50 mL.（2 amp 左右）

        C. 起始 10–20 mins，peaks at 30–60 mins，持續 4–6 hours，效果：K^+ ↓ 0.5–1.2 mmol/L。

        D. 小心低血糖。75% 病人在接受 bolus regimen 後一小時左右發生。

    (2) β-agonist：建議和 insulin/glucose 合用

        A. 起始 30 mins, peaks at 90 mins, 持續 2–6 hours，效果：K^+ ↓ 0.5–1.0 mmol/L。

        B. Synergism with insulin 且可減少低血糖的發生。

        C. 20%–40% of ESRD patients NOT responsive to albuterol. β2-agonists should not be used as a single agent to treat hyperkalemia.

(3) Bicarbonate: Controversial

   Suggested ONLY in acidemia

4. 增加鉀從身體裡排出

   (1) Diuretics，尤其是在 hyporeninemic hypoaldosteronism 的狀況，或有 K$^+$ secretory problems。

   (2) 交換樹脂 (resins)，效果很慢（頭 24 hours 幾無作用），要避開服用其他陽離子。常見 K$^+$ 交換樹脂有以下四種，其中 patiromer 和 zirconium 為比較新的選擇，其特性可參考 Table 4-6 [6]：

   A. Kayexalate/Kuzem (sodium polystyrene sulfonate): Na$^+$-cycled resins
   → Na$^+$ 吸收增加，小心 volume overload。

   B. Kalimate: calcium-cycled resins
   → 小心 hypercalcemia，此外也可能降磷。

   C. Patiromer: patiromer sorbitex calcium (Veltassa)

   D. Zirconium: sodium zirconium cyclosilicate (Lokelma [formerly ZS-9])

   (3) Dialysis，最快最有效，但也最具侵入性風險最大

   A. 3–5 hr 的 hemodialysis 可移除 40–120 mmoL 的鉀，其中第一小時是移除最多最快的，第三小時後移除量就很有限了

   B. 血鉀和透析液落差太大，降鉀太快可能會增加 arrhythmia 和反彈性高血壓的風險，尤其在老人、有吃 digoxin、病史有 arrhythmia、coronary artery disease、left ventricular hypertrophy、high systolic blood pressure 者。

   C. Pre-treatment with β2-agonist, insulin and glucose, 或透析中吃東西會減少鉀被移除的效率（因為躲進細胞內），造成透析後 K$^+$ 升高

5. Treatment of underlying conditions 以及飲食和藥物調整。

Table 4-6. 鉀交換樹脂的比較 [a]

	Cation exchange resin	Patiromer	SZC
商品名	• Kayexalate, Kuzem (Na^+ polystyrene sulfonate) • Kalimate (Ca^{2+} polystyrene sulfonate)	Veltassa	Lokelma
核准日期	1958	美國，2015；歐盟，2017	美國，2018；歐盟，2018
作用機轉	於腸胃道內以 Na^+ 或 Ca^{2+} 交換 K^+，增加糞便 K^+ 排除量	於腸胃道內結合 K^+ 並交換 Ca^{2+}	於腸胃道內結合 K^+ 並交換 Na^+ 和 H^+
作用位置	大腸	大腸	小腸及大腸
對 K^+ 的選擇性	• 無選擇性；也會結合其他陽離子（Na^+, Ca^{2+}, Mg^{2+}） • Kayexalate: 每 g 約可結合 1 mEq K^+ • Kalimate: 每 g 約可結合 1.36–1.82 mEq Na^+	無選擇性；也會結合 Na^+ 和 Mg^{2+}	高度選擇性；但也結合 NH_4^+
開始作用的時間	Variable; several hours	7 hr	1 hr
Na^+ 含量	Kayexalate, Kuzem 每 g 約含 4.1 mEq Na^+	無	每 5 g 中含 400 mg Na^+
Ca^{2+} 含量	Kalimate 含 7%–9% Ca^{2+}	每 8.4 g 中含 1.6 g Ca^{2+}	無
山梨糖醇 (sorbitol) 含量	無	每 8.4 g 中含 4,000 mg Sorbitol	無
劑量	• Kayexalate, Kuzem：每天 15 g 1–4 次（口服）；30 g 1–2 次（經直腸） • Kalimate：每天 5–10 g 2–3 次（口服）；每次 30 g，留置 30–60 min（經直腸）	每天 8.4 g（口服），可慢慢增加到每天 16.8 g 或 25.2 g	剛開始降鉀的急性期：每天 10 g 3 次（口服）（不超過 48 hr） 維持期：每兩天 5 g 到每天 15 g
嚴重副作用	當與山梨糖醇（sorbitol）一起給予時，有報告指出會造成致命的腸胃道損傷（缺血性大腸炎）	無相關報告	無相關報告
常見的副作用	• 共通副作用：腸胃不適（便祕、拉肚子、噁心、嘔吐、胃部不適） • Kayexalate, Kuzem：低血鎂、低血鉀、低血鈣、水份滯留 • Kalimate：低血鉀、高血鈣	腸胃不適（便祕、拉肚子、噁心、脹氣）、低血鎂（9%）	腸胃不適（便祕、拉肚子、噁心、嘔吐）、輕至中度水腫

Abbreviation: SZC, sodium zirconium cyclosilicate.

[a] 資料參考來源：[6]。

參考文獻

[1] Bhat P, Dretler A, Gdowski M, Ramgopal R, Williams D. *The Washington Manual of Medical Therapeutics*. 35th ed. Philadelphia, PA: Wolters Kluwer; 2016.

[2] Ellison DH, Berl T. Clinical practice. The syndrome of inappropriate antidiuresis. *N Engl J Med*. 2007;356(20):2064-2072. doi:10.1056/NEJMcp066837

[3] Adrogué HJ, Madias NE. Hyponatremia. *N Engl J Med*. 2000;342(21):1581-1589. doi:10.1056/NEJM200005253422107

[4] 李忠政，黃文德，林石化。低血鉀的診斷與治療。內科學誌。2011；22(1)：31-39。doi:10.6314/JIMT.2011.22(1).04

[5] Yu ASL, Chertow G, Luyckx V, Marsden P, Skorecki K, Taal M, eds. *Brenner and Rector's The Kidney*. 11th ed. Philadelphia, PA: Elsevier; 2020.

[6] Palmer BF. Potassium binders for hyperkalemia in chronic kidney disease-diet, renin-angiotensin-aldosterone system inhibitor therapy, and hemodialysis. *Mayo Clin Proc*. 2020;95(2):339-354. doi:10.1016/j.mayocp.2019.05.019

延伸閱讀文獻

李忠政，黃文德，林石化。低血鉀的診斷與治療。內科學誌。2011；22(1)：31-39。doi:10.6314/JIMT.2011.22(1).04

Adrogué HJ, Madias NE. Hyponatremia. *N Engl J Med*. 2000;342(21):1581-1589. doi:10.1056/NEJM200005253422107

Arroyo JP, Ronzaud C, Lagnaz D, Staub O, Gamba G. Aldosterone paradox: differential regulation of ion transport in distal nephron. *Physiology (Bethesda)*. 2011;26(2):115-123. doi:10.1152/physiol.00049.2010

Bhat P, Dretler A, Gdowski M, Ramgopal R, Williams D. *The Washington Manual of Medical Therapeutics*. 35th ed. Philadelphia, PA: Wolters Kluwer; 2016.

New South Wales Government, Northern Sydney Local Health District. Intravenous potassium chloride guideline (adult)-NSRHS. https://vdocuments.mx/intravenous-potassium-chloride-guideline.html?page=1. Published April 30, 2014.

Palmer BF. Potassium binders for hyperkalemia in chronic kidney disease-diet, renin-angiotensin-aldosterone system inhibitor therapy, and hemodialysis. *Mayo Clin Proc*. 2020;95(2):339-354. doi:10.1016/j.mayocp.2019.05.019

Sabatine MS. *Pocket Medicine: The Massachusetts General Hospital Handbook of Internal Medicine*. 7th ed. Philadelphia, PA: Wolters Kluwer Health; 2019.

Yu ASL, Chertow G, Luyckx V, Marsden P, Skorecki K, Taal M, eds. *Brenner and Rector's The Kidney*. 11th ed. Philadelphia, PA: Elsevier; 2020.

Chapter 5

Laboratory Assessment of Renal Function by Blood and Urine

李宗翰
臺北榮民總醫院腎臟科

蔡明村
臺北榮民總醫院腎臟科

腎功能異常不易被發現，症狀出現時往往已是疾病晚期，因此臨床醫師需要借助常規血液和尿液的檢驗，協助早期發現腎功能異常病人及後續追蹤監控。

一、常見腎功能之血液指標

（一）血清尿素氮 (Blood Urea Nitrogen, BUN)

　　尿素是蛋白質代謝的終端產物，在肝臟合成後，進入血液循環而由腎臟排泄。在體液中尿素能自由進出細胞內外及微血管壁，尿素經腎絲球濾過後，40% 到 50% 在腎小管（大部分在近曲小管）被再吸收，若病患身體處於脫水狀態，近曲小管增加對水和鈉離子再吸收時，會同時增加對尿素氮的再吸收，換言之，BUN 可能在腎臟灌流不足時不成比例的升高。因此，臨床上常以計算尿素氮和肌酸酐 (creatinine) 的比值，藉此評估腎前疾病的可能性。Table 5-1 列出影響 BUN/Cr 比值的各種情形。

　　BUN 的濃度通常是由：1. 每天攝食蛋白質的總量，以及體內蛋白質異化作用所產生的尿素和 2. 腎臟排泄尿素的速率等二個因素所決定；由於蛋白質的攝食量及尿液排泄量每人差異很大，其在血中的濃度正常值為 8–18 mg/dL。測得較低的尿素氮濃度可能意味著低蛋白質攝取或慢性肝臟疾病（因為合成速率下降）；反之，當腎功能明顯障礙時，BUN 濃度會顯著上升，但也可能因為其他非腎臟因素上升，例如：增加蛋白質的攝取、腸胃道出血（因為腸胃道從血液成分中吸收氨基酸），或使用皮質類固醇時導致身體處於高異化代謝狀態等。

　　綜上所述，由於 BUN 會受到太多非腎絲球過濾率 (glomeruler filtration rate, GFR) 因素影響，其較難成為評估腎臟功能 (GFR) 的獨立生物指標，需同時參考其他指標和病患的臨床表現才能做完整的判讀。

（二）血清肌酸酐 (Serum Creatinine, SCr)

　　肌酸 (creatine) 在肝臟合成之後，以游離型及磷肌酸 (phosphocreatine) 的形式大量存在於肌肉組織，磷肌酸提供肌肉使用三磷酸腺苷後的磷酸補充。肌酸藉由 creatine phosphokinase 的催化，轉變成脫水產物肌酸酐。每天肌酸轉換成肌酸酐的比率大抵是恆定的（約 2%）。血液裡的肌酸酐經過腎絲球的過濾及腎小管的分泌作用排出體外，每天尿液中排出的肌酸酐總量視肌肉組織的多少而定，相對來說比較不會受到蛋白質攝食量或尿量變動的影響，但會與年齡、性別、種族、身體組成、身形大小、活動度、肌肉是否受傷（如橫紋肌溶解）有關。腎小管會分泌肌酸酐且再吸收甚少，當肌酸酐的分泌受到藥物（如：trimethoprim、cimetidine）抑制或腎功能減損時，血中的肌酸

酐值會上升。當肌酸酐的分泌因為腎病症候群抑制或鐮刀型貧血等疾病上升時，血中的肌酸酐值可能下降。正常人血中的肌酸酐值大致維持在 0.6–1.5 mg/dL。

（三）血中尿素氮和肌酸酐比值 (Serum BUN to Cr Ratio, BUN/Cr)

在正常的腎臟功能下，血中尿素氮和肌酸酐比值約為 10:1。當身體發生下列情形時，會造成此比值的上升或下降（Table 5-1）：

（四）Cystatin C

Cystatin C 越來越常用在臨床作為腎功能評估的指標，它是一種小分子量蛋白，它在腎絲球被濾過後不會被再吸收，然而，它可能被腎小管代謝。有一些非腎功能因素可能影響 Cystatin C 的血清濃度，例如，男性、身高較高、體重較重、糖尿病、發炎指標高、甲狀腺亢進或低下、使用類固醇等因素會使 Cystatin C 濃度上升，且一樣有年紀及種族間的差異。

二、常見腎功能之尿液指標

（一）尿液分析 (Urinalysis)

每日尿液約為 1,200–1,500 mL，取得容易。晨起第一泡尿在傳統上是最好的檢體且和連續 24 小時尿液收集檢體有較好的相關，較不會受到飲食、飲水、姿勢、運動等

Table 5-1. 影響身體 BUN/Cr 比值的各種情形

Serum BUN to Cr ratio	症狀
BUN/Cr > 10:1	腎臟血流量減少：血管內體液不足、利尿劑、心衰竭等。
	增加尿素氮合成：蛋白質攝取、腸胃道出血、四環黴素、發燒、使用類固醇、外傷、敗血症、組織壞死等。
	腸胃道吸收上升：感染、腎衰竭、外傷等。
BUN/Cr < 10:1	尿素氮下降：酒精成癮、慢性肝病、營養不良等。
	肌酸酐上升：Trimethoprim、cimetidine 等藥物會抑制腎小管分泌肌酸酐。
	Acetoacetate（DKA 時）、Bilirubin、Cefoxitin、Flucytosine 會影響測量肌酸酐的準確度。
	橫紋肌溶解症。

Abbreviations: BUN, blood urea nitrogen; Cr, creatinine; DKA, diabetic ketoacidosis.

的因素影響，且濃縮呈酸性可以保存較好。臨床操作上收集 24 小時尿液較不方便，故常利用單次尿液作為檢體。尿液分析包括物理性檢查，利用尿液試紙的化學性檢查，以及尿沉渣顯微檢查。

1. 物理性檢查

(1) 外觀清澈度：受尿液中白血球、細菌、紅血球 (red blood cell, RBC)、結晶、黏液等物質之多寡影響。

(2) 顏色：紅色尿表示尿中帶有血色素 (hemoglobin)、肌紅蛋白 (myoglobin) 或藥物、食物造成；黃褐色尿表示尿中含鐵物質、高膽紅素 (hyperbilirubin) 等；白色尿表示尿中可能含淋巴液、膿、磷酸結晶等。

(3) 泡沫：小便至馬桶或小便後沖水至馬桶出現泡沫，且要沖水 2–3 次，泡沫才會消失，表示尿中可能含有超過正常量之蛋白。

(4) 尿比重 (specific gravity)：

檢測範圍值為 1.001–1.035。尿比重的高低與血液的 osmolarity 大致成正相關。當體內水分不足時，尿比重會上升；尿中酸鹼值 (pH) 小於 6 時會假性偏高，尿中酸鹼值大於 7 時則會假性偏低。因腎臟之濃縮能力隨年齡上升而減弱，尿比重也會隨年齡上升而下降。

2. 化學性檢查

(1) 尿液酸鹼值 (pH)：正常值為 4.5–8.5，會受食物、身體狀況及藥物影響。肉類、水果（如小紅莓等）、酸血症、體液不足等會使 pH 值下降。素食、柑橘類水果、鹼血症、第一型腎小管酸血症等，會使尿液酸鹼值上升。

(2) 尿蛋白 (proteinuria)：尿液試紙中的試劑對白蛋白敏銳度遠高於其他蛋白質，因此當尿中有其他球蛋白、血色素或游離輕鍵 (light chain)，測試結果可能為偽陰性。依尿蛋白量之多少可分為微量 (5–20 mg/dL)、1＋(30 mg/dL)、2＋(100 mg/dL)、3＋(300 mg/dL) 和 4＋(＞1,000 mg/dL)。若尿液試紙檢查中，尿蛋白呈陰性或微量，但定量的尿蛋白肌酸酐比值卻為陽性或強陽性，則表示尿中含有異常的球蛋白，必須進一步做檢查，以確認病患是否患有多發性骨髓瘤等血液疾病。

(3) 尿潛血 (occult blood)：尿液試紙可以驗出含鐵物質。當潛血反應呈陽性而尿沉渣檢查中 RBC 呈陰性時，要注意病患是否出現溶血或橫紋肌溶解症；此時必須檢查周邊血液抹片，測量血中乳酸脫氫酶 (lactate dehydrogenase)、血色素結合蛋白 (haptoglobin) 及血清肌酸磷酸脢 (creatinine kinase) 以確定病因。

(4) 尿糖 (urine glucose)：較血糖不準。尿量會影響數值。尿糖較血糖晚上升因此只能限制用於篩檢。一旦測出尿糖通常表示血糖超過 210 mg/dL。

(5) 尿酮 (ketones)：正常尿液中不會檢出 β-hydroxybutyrate（酮酸血症中占全部血清酮酸的 80%）。若病人有服用 ascorbic acid 和 phenazopyridine 等藥物時會造成尿酮偽陽性，需進一步測血清酮酸以確認。

(6) 尿膽紅素 (bilirubin) 及尿膽原 (urobilinogen)：只有直接型膽紅素會排至尿中，所以阻塞型黃疸和肝細胞受損時，尿膽紅素會呈陽性，而溶血造成的黃疸，尿膽紅素呈陰性，尿膽原呈陽性；若尿液遭糞便染污、尿液檢體儲存過久或遭光線照射等，尿膽紅素會呈偽陽性。

(7) 亞硝酸鹽 (nitrite)：革蘭氏陰性腸內菌經常是造成尿道炎的主要原因。較常見是 *Escherichia coli*，比較不常見如 *Proteus*、*Enterobacter*、*Klebsiella* 等菌含有 nitrate reductase（記法：PECK），會將 urine 中的 nitrate 還原成 nitrite。尿中菌需花四小時才能將硝酸鹽轉變為亞硝酸 (nitrite)。不會轉換此過程的菌種有：腸球菌屬 (*Enterococcus*, e.g., *E. faecalis*)、*Neisseria gonorrhoeae* 和結核菌。膀胱滯留時間不夠久會偽陰性。但如果檢體儲存太久會導致亞硝酸裂解也會偽陰性。

3. 尿沉渣顯微檢查 (Urine Sediment Microscopic Examinations)

主要在顯微鏡下觀察尿液中所含之沉渣物質，常見之尿沉渣如下：

(1) RBC：主要是源自腎間質或泌尿道上皮，高倍鏡下超過 2 個 RBCs 即被視為異常。但在發燒，生理期，運動後，尿中也可出現較多的 RBCs。

(2) 白血球：高倍鏡下超過 5 個白血球，被視為異常。最常見原因是泌尿道感染，也可能是間質性腎炎 (interstitial nephritis)、急性腎絲球腎炎、腎移植後急性排斥反應或造成泌尿道周圍發炎反應的腸胃炎或急性盲腸炎。

(3) 嗜伊紅性白血球：暗示過敏性間質腎炎，需了解病人的用藥或食物史，儘快找出造成過敏之原因。

(4) 上皮細胞：尿液中出現大量腎小管上皮細胞 (tubular cells) 可能原因為急性腎小管壞死、間質性腎炎或腎移植後急性排斥反應等。若是大量泌尿道上皮細胞 (transitional epithelial cells)，則可能原因為感染、腫瘤或結石。

(5) 圓柱體 (casts) 及結晶 (crystals) (Table 5-2)。

（二）血尿 (Hematuria)

1. 定義

正常人平均一天尿液中 RBCs 有 1,000,000 個，每毫升尿液可達 5,000–10,000 個 RBCs，相當於尿液檢查高倍鏡下 1–2 個 RBCs，所以當尿沉渣在高倍鏡下出現超過 2 個 RBCs 時，被定義為血尿。

Table 5-2. 尿液中常見之圓柱體或結晶，在臨床上可能代表之意義 [a]

類型	臨床代表意義
圓柱體	紅血球：腎絲球腎炎
	白血球：急性間質腎炎、急性腎盂腎炎、腎絲球腎炎顆粒 (granular: muddy brown)、急性間質腎炎。
	腎小管上皮細胞：急性腎小管壞死
	玻璃質 (hyaline)：主要內容物為 Tamm-Horsfall protein，當腎臟疾病、心衰竭或發燒時，其尿中數量會增加。
	Waxy and broad：晚期腎衰竭
晶體	一水草酸鈣 (calcium oxalate monohydrate)：針狀、卵圓狀、啞鈴型
	二水草酸鈣 (calcium oxalate dihydrate)：六面稜鏡型
	尿酸 (uric acid: variable shape)：偏極光下呈多色
	胱胺酸 (cystine)：六角型
	鳥糞石／磷酸銨鎂 (struvite)：coffin-lid，會分解尿素的菌種造成的慢性泌尿道感染

[a] 資料參考來源：[1]

2. 血尿與色素尿 (Pigmenturia) 如何分別

(1) 血尿為紅或紅褐色尿液，且尿沉渣在高倍鏡下出現超過 2 個 RBCs。

(2) 色素尿是因食物，藥物（如結核藥），或疾病（如：紫質症 porphyria、溶血、外傷、燒傷、橫紋肌溶解症、瓣膜等植入物）會造成尿液呈現紅或紅褐色，但尿沉渣中 RBC 為陰性，必須尋找原因，加以治療。

3. 血尿原因

很多如腎絲球腎炎、血管、感染、結石、腫瘤、外傷、藥物、代謝遺傳家族史等。生理性原因，如發燒、運動、長途賽跑等也會引起血尿。各年齡層有其好發原因，成人最常見原因為腎絲球腎炎、泌尿道感染、結石、腫瘤、攝護腺肥大、高鈣尿症和高尿酸尿症等。結石和泌尿道感染各年齡都有，惡性腫瘤和攝護腺肥大則隨著年齡上升增加。

4. 血尿鑑別診斷

分顯微血尿或巨觀血尿，源自腎絲球或非源自腎絲球。源自腎絲球的血尿者會有 RBC 圓柱體、重度蛋白尿、大量變形紅血球 (dysmorphic RBCs) 等特徵 (Figure 5-1)。

（三）蛋白尿 (Proteinuria)

1. 每天血液經過腎臟濾出的蛋白質大約有 11,000–14,000 g，較小的蛋白質 (< 20 KDa) 可被動穿過微血管而濾出，低分子量蛋白會在近端腎小管再吸收，所以非常少量 α2-

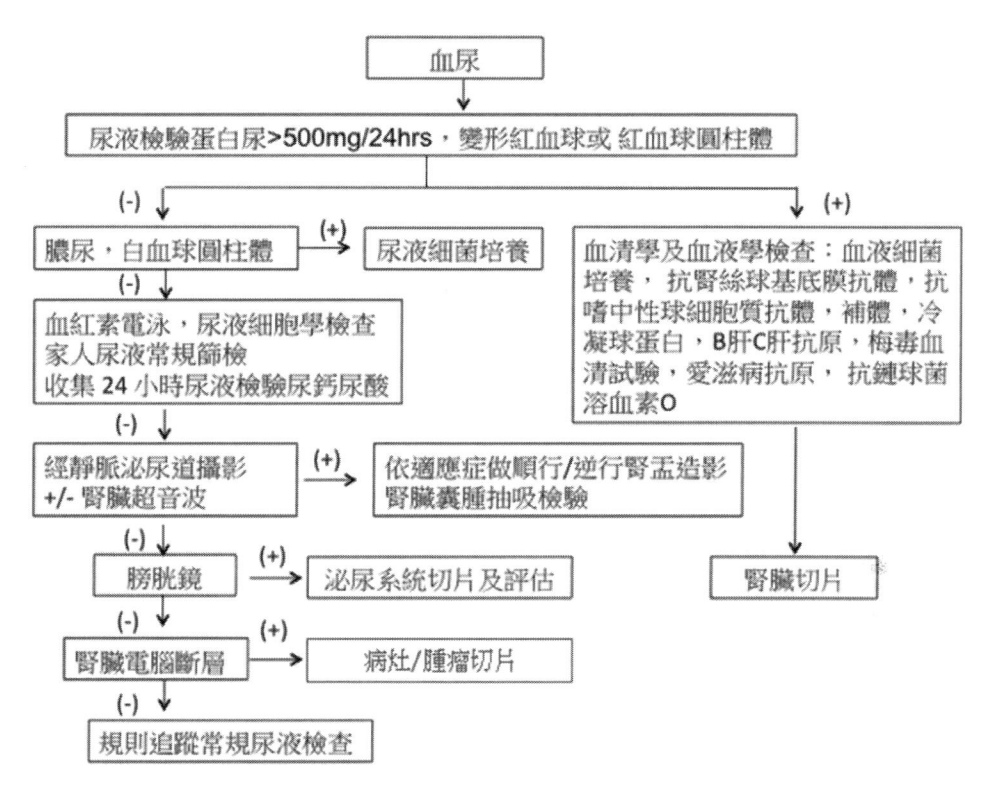

Figure 5-1. 血尿之評估流程 [a]

[a] 資料參考來源：[2]。

microglobulin、apoproteins、酵素和肽類激素 (peptide hormones) 會出現在尿液裡。尿蛋白中白蛋白占 30%–40%，immunoglobulin G (IgG) 占 5%–10%，light chains 5%，IgA 3%。尿蛋白正常約為 40–80 mg，上限為每天 200 mg，正常尿中不會出現高分子量蛋白，如 IgD、IgM 等。

2. 定性測量方式：尿試紙檢驗

尿液試紙上浸潤 pH 指示染劑 (tetrabromophenol blue)，原理是根據蛋白質多寡改變試紙顏色，顏色改變從黃到藍的程度大致上與蛋白質濃度呈正相關。鹼性尿、濃縮尿、巨觀血尿會造成尿試紙蛋白檢驗呈偽陽性；稀釋尿，則可能會造成尿試紙蛋白檢驗呈偽陰性。

3. 定量測量方式

測量尿中每天的蛋白總量可經由 24 小時尿液收集（不方便，容易因收集過程有誤差）或單次尿液尿蛋白質／肌酸酐比值 (spot urine protein/creatinine) 來測量 24 小時的尿蛋白量（公式如下）。原理是利用蛋白質與 trichloroacetic acid 或 sulfosalicylic acid 產生沉澱作用，使用濁度計定量。此方法可使輕鏈產生沉澱而測得陽性並定量。正常值是小於 200 mg/g。

$$\frac{\text{Uprot}}{\text{Ucrea}} = \frac{\text{Upro} \times \text{V}}{\text{Ucrea} \times \text{V}} = \frac{\text{24 hours urine protein}}{\text{24 hours urine creatinine}}$$

(1) 尿蛋白量的高低可作為診斷及預後的參考：當腎絲球病變引起微血管屏障破壞時，會濾出大量大分子量蛋白質如白蛋白，通常可以一天超過 3 g。例如腎絲球腎炎、腎病症候群等。若腎小管受損使近端腎小管回收蛋白質能力下降時，尿中小分子量蛋白質增加，且很少一天超過 2 g，如 Fanconi's syndrome、急性腎小管壞死和急性間質腎炎等。

(2) 當身體製造大量可被腎絲球濾過的蛋白質或是病態不應存在的蛋白質量超過腎小管可以回收的負荷時，蛋白就會隨著尿液排出。若尿中增加的是單一種輕鍵，比較像是增加蛋白質合成，當尿中增加的是混合 kappa 和 lambda 不同輕鍵，則可能是源發自腎小管的疾病。正常來說每天只有排出 3 mg 輕鍵且 kappa/lambda 所占比值約為 3。不過製造過多時，尿蛋白一天可以高達 15 g。此類疾病包括多發性骨髓瘤、heavy-chain disease、macroglobulinemia、idiopathic light-chain proteinuria、外傷造成肌紅蛋白尿、溶血造成血色素尿等。

(3) 功能性白蛋白尿：正常人在激烈運動後會有短暫 2–3 倍上升的蛋白尿，通常運動結束後幾小時會回復正常。其它像是發燒、嚴重情緒壓力、心衰竭等都有可能出現短暫蛋白尿。

(4) 姿勢性白蛋白尿：慢性腎臟病病人在站立姿勢時蛋白尿會增加。量通常不會超過 1 g，目前認為是良性的情況。可分兩個時段收集尿液，一是白天有日常活動的 16 小時，另一是睡眠的 8 小時，比較兩個時段蛋白尿的差別可知是否有姿勢性白蛋白尿。

4. 如何分析蛋白尿（見 Figure 5-2）

第一步是用尿液試紙檢查看是否有白蛋白尿。若為陽性則可能為腎絲球病變所產生之蛋白尿；如果陰性，則可能是腎小管病變或腎間質腎炎，或身體製造大量病態不應存在的蛋白質。下一步就是要做 electrophoresis 或其他檢查方法以確認蛋白尿原因。

三、腎功能之監控與追蹤

臨床上常使用血液及尿液之腎功能指標，做為腎功能變化及治療效果的參考，但腎元的數目隨年紀遞減，因此正常腎功能隨年紀性別有所不同，45 歲以下 GFR 每年下降 0.4 mL/min/1.73m^2，45 歲之後則每年下降 0.75 mL/min/1.73m^2。所以在測量腎功能 (GFR) 時，需要用體表面積及年紀來做校正，臨床上並因此而利用上述指標發展更敏

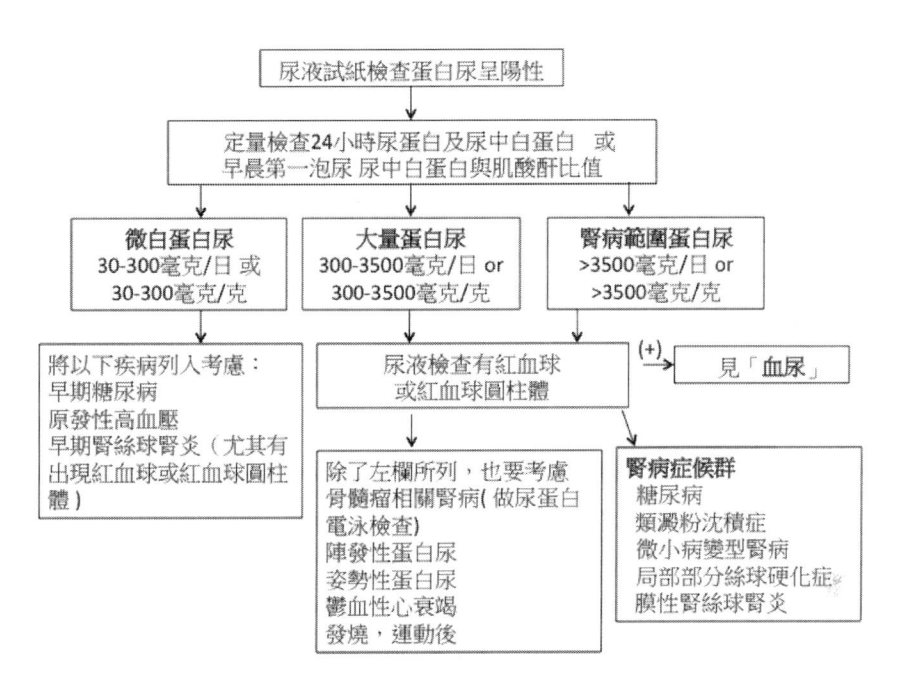

Figure 5-2. 蛋白尿之評估 [a]

[a] 資料參考來源：[2]。

感之公式來估算腎功能，作為腎功能長期監控追蹤的參考。常用之公式包含 Cockcroft-Gault equation (C-G equation)、chronic kidney disease epidemiology collaboration (CKD-EPI) equation 以及 modification of diet in renal disease (MDRD) study equation，其中，CKD-EPI equation 和 MDRD equation 有用體表面積作校正，其準確程度優於 C-G equation，這些公式的介紹如下：

（一）C-G Equation

$$CrCl(mL/min) = \frac{(140 - Age) \times body\ weight[kg]}{Cr\left[\frac{mg}{dL}\right] \times 72} \times 0.85(If\ female)$$

此公式將年紀變大肌酸酐生成量會下降、體重較重肌酸酐生成量較大等因素納入考量，然而，這個公式發展的時代，肥胖並未如現今般普遍，在沒有校正體表面積的情況下，經常高估肥胖或水腫病人會高估 GFR。然而，因為簡單方便計算，且許多藥物動力學決定劑量之臨床試驗（如抗生素）大多用此公式評估 GFR。因此，此公式仍在臨床應用上占有一席之地，用於評估 SCr 兩週內呈穩定狀態病患之腎功能。

（二）MDRD Study Equation

$$GFR[mL/min \times 1.73m^2] = 175 \times SCr(exp[-1.154]) \times Age(exp[-0.203]) \times (0.742 \text{ if female}) \times (1.21 \text{ if Black})$$

Note: MDRD 公式之常數 175 適用於 isotope dilution mass spectrometry (IDMS)-traceable assay 測定之 SCr 值。若 SCr 值非由經 IDMS 校正者，此常數應改為 186。

此公式源自於收錄進 MDRD 試驗的病患資料，其病患資料擴及多種族（白種人、非裔美洲人、歐洲人、亞洲人）及多種腎臟疾病，對於慢性穩定病患相較於 C-G 公式有較高的準確率，尤其是在老年人和肥胖的患者。然而，因為運算時使用參數比較多，使用上較為困難。腎功能較好的病人容易低估 GFR，在 eGFR > 60 mL/min/1.73 m² 較不適用。

（三）CKD-EPI Equation

$$eGFR_{cr-cys} = 135 \times \min\left(\frac{Scr}{\kappa}, 1\right)^{\alpha} \times \max\left(\frac{Scr}{\kappa}, 1\right)^{-0.544} \times \min\left(\frac{Scys}{0.8}, 1\right)^{-0.323} \\ \times \max\left(\frac{Scys}{0.8}, 1\right)^{-0.778} \times 0.9961^{Age} \times 0.963(\text{if female})$$

κ = 0.7(female) or 0.9(male)
α = -0.219(female) or -0.144(male)

此公式發展源於 2009 年，目的在更精確的評估正常或僅有些微減損 GFR 的族群，其蒐集來自超過 20 個臨床研究的資料，證實其對於 eGFR < 60 mL/min 之病患，有和 MDRD 相仿的準確率，對於 eGFR > 60 mL/min 之病患有更好的準確率。2021 年，CKD-EPI 發表了新的計算公式，此公式的發展除了原本 2009 年的資料，又納入了額外超過 10 個臨床研究的病患資料，此公式不再加入種族為參數，雖然其準確度稍差一點點，但應用於臨床已相當足夠。2021 CKD-EPI creatinine-cystatin C equation 結合 creatinine 和 cystatin C 作為計算參數，比僅用 creatinine 或僅用 cystatin C 都較準確。

（四）24-Hour Urine Creatinine Clearance (CCr)

$$24 \text{ hours CCr(mL/min)} = \frac{\text{Urine creatinine(mg/dL)} \times 24 \text{ hours urine volume(mL)}}{\text{Serum creatinine(mg/dL)} \times 1440 \text{ mins}}$$

此法優點為不被身體肌肉含量影響，缺點為尿液不易正確收集執行。

四、結論

　　雖然有各種腎功能的估算公式，但沒有一種公式可以精準套用到所有不同腎功能的病人，最客觀之估算方法為同一病人持續定期的監測，自己和自己之前的數據相比。臨床上常使用上述血液及尿液指標作為腎功能之監測，優點是方便便宜，缺點是腎損傷初期不會立即升高；因腎小管在腎絲球受損時還保有主動分泌的能力。腎臟功能的測定是非常簡單的，只要我們從血液的 BUN、肌酸酐、尿液的常規檢查、肌酸酐、尿量及尿蛋白，再加上年齡指標，可看出病人在其年齡層是否有異常，同時使用這些公式在同一病人身上作追蹤，則可進一步看出腎功能的變化情形，作為臨床判斷治療的參考。

參考文獻

[1] Sabatine MS, ed. *Pocket Medicine: The Massachusetts General Hospital Handbook of Internal Medicine*. 5th ed. Philadelphia, PA: Lippincott Williams and Wilkins; 2013.

[2] Jameson JL, Fauci AS, Kasper DL, Hauser SL, Longo DL, Loscalzo J, eds. *Harrison's Principles of Internal Medicine*. 20th ed. New York, NY: McGraw Hill; 2018.

延伸閱讀文獻

Inker LA, Lafayette LA, Upadhyay A, Levey AS. Laboratory evaluation of kidney disease. In: Schrier RW, Coffman TM, Falk RJ, Molitoris BA, Neilson EG, eds. *Schrier's Diseases of the Kidney*. 9th ed. Philadelphia, PA: Lippincott Williams and Wilkins; 2012:295-345.

Inker LA, Perrone RD. Assessment of kidney function. UpToDate Web site. https://www.uptodate.com/contents/assessment-of-kidney-function. Updated March 14, 2023.

Jameson JL, Fauci AS, Kasper DL, Hauser SL, Longo DL, Loscalzo J, eds. *Harrison's Principles of Internal Medicine*. 20th ed. New York, NY: McGraw Hill; 2018.

Parikh CR, Koyner JL. Biomarkers in acute and chronic kidney diseases. In: Yu ASL, Chertow GM, Luyckx V, Marsden PA, Skorecki K, Taal MW, eds. *Brenner and Rector's The Kidney*. 11th ed. Philadelphia, PA: Elsevier; 2019:872-904.

Chapter 6

Imaging: Diagnostic Characteristics of Common Kidney Diseases

蔡友蓮
臺北榮民總醫院腎臟科

曾偉誠
臺北榮民總醫院腎臟科

沈書慧
臺北榮民總醫院放射線部

隨著科技發展的日新月異，醫學影像系統取得了重大的進展，協助我們瞭解內在器官系統的結構功能。X 光片主要提供解剖訊息，包含靜脈尿路攝影 (intravenous urography)，順型和逆行性腎盂顯影 (antegrade and retrograde pyelography)。其他影像檢查工具包含電腦斷層 (computed tomography, CT)、超音波與核子醫學影像等。瞭解每種檢查成像方式、診斷效用和局限性將有助於在各種特定臨床環境中對患者進行正確評估。

一、超音波 (Ultrasonography)

由於超音波檢查方便簡單，價格便宜，無輻射性和侵入性，因此常是腎臟疾病的首選檢查。不同的組織具有不同的聲阻抗 (acoustic impedance)。當聲波穿過不同的組織時，部分聲波被反射回探頭 (transducer)，便可藉聲波返回探頭的時間來測量組織界面的深度。探頭所接收之反射聲波經由電腦轉換成灰階圖像，其像素的強度與反射聲波的強度成正比，如骨骼、脂肪和纖維組織會反射大部分聲波，為高回音性 (hyperechoic)，呈現亮白色 (bright white)。骨骼和空氣對於聲音的強烈反射導致其下方組織無法接收與反射聲波，進而無法顯現下方組織，此現象稱為聲音陰影 (acoustic shadowing)。在充滿液體的結構（例如膀胱和腎囊腫 [cyst]）中由於聲波可以輕鬆穿過，使遠端的強度相對增加；這被稱為遠端回音增強 (distal acoustic enhancement)。這些特徵都可用於鑑別各種病變。

都卜勒超音波 (Doppler ultrasonography)，原理是透過物體移動時引起聲波頻率改變（頻移，frequency shift）移動，可以用於評估靜脈和動脈的血流。當探頭持續向血管發射聲波，因血管內的血球為流動之物體，故移動之血球所反射之聲波便產生頻移。當血球朝向聲波源（探頭）移動時，反射波波長被壓縮而頻率增加；反之血球遠聲波源時，反射波波長變長而頻率減少。反射波頻率變化量則與血液流速成正比，因而彩色都卜勒超音波可將反射波頻率之增加或減少以紅色或藍色顯示，頻移變化量則以不同顏色亮度呈現。

阻力指數 (resistant index, RI) 是腎臟內動脈血流阻力的指標，定義為：（收縮期峰值速度 [peak systolic velocity] – 舒張末期速度 [end diastolic velocity]）/ 收縮期峰值速度 (peak systolic velocity)，正常範圍是 0.50–0.70。高 RI (> 0.8) 與非移植腎臟病之腎功能不良與心血管事件增加有相關，亦與腎移植病人之移植腎失去功能或死亡有相關。

一般腎臟在超音波下有以下特點：高音波反射的結構或病徵，例如腎包膜 (renal capsule) 或結石 (stone)，會呈現亮白色高回音性影像，且會在病灶後方造成黑暗的 distal shadow。而如果是含液體的病灶，例如腎囊腫，則會呈現 hypoechoic（黑暗的）影像，但在病灶後方會顯示加強的回音性 (echogenicity)，即 distal enhancement。而像是 renal parenchyma 的回音性則是介於中間。

腎臟的超音波影像通常呈現的方式為縱向 (longitudinal)、橫向 (transverse/axial) 和矢狀面 (sagittal)。正常成人的腎臟包含許多腎葉 (lobe)，每個腎葉皆由一個腎髓質錐體 (medullary pyramid) 與其上之皮質 (cortex rim) 所構成，其會在終端形成腎乳頭 (papilla) 並突出延伸進入小腎盞 (minor calyx)。在兩個腎錐體中間的皮質稱為 Bertin 式柱 (column of Bertin)。小腎盞會匯集形成大腎盞 (major calyx)，並最終形成腎盂 (renal pelvis) (Figure 6-1)。腎臟中非腎實質 (parenchyma) 也非尿腔 (urinary space) 的地方則稱為腎竇 (renal sinus)。成人腎竇在會被脂肪組織充滿，因此呈現 hyperechoic。腎竇的脂肪量通常隨著年齡的增長而增加。

在超音波縱向面下，正常腎臟呈現卵形，與肝臟和脾臟相比，正常的腎皮質回音性較弱（即看起來更暗）。腎臟中間是 hyperechoic (bright) central sinus，其外圍則為 hypoechoic (dark) rim of cortex 和 medulla。回音性由高至低排序是 renal sinus > liver/spleen > renal cortex > renal pyramid (medulla)。對應於血管和集尿系統的管狀結構在腎門 (hilum) 中可見。都卜勒彩色超音波可用於區分血管和集尿系統。

正常成人腎臟約 10–12 cm 長。腎臟長度和身高成正比，且取決於年齡性別和體質。腎臟的輪廓是光滑的。從腎門到主動脈和下腔靜脈 (inferior vena cava)，可以看到腎動脈和腎靜脈。靜脈位於動脈前面。懷孕時腎臟會因為 parenchymal enlargement 而變大，並在生產後 12 週後回復正常大小。由於正常腎臟位於背側，因此最好是請病患趴臥 (prone position)，從後方檢查，可得到較清楚的影像 (Figure 6-2)。

如果在正常位置未發現腎臟，則應評估腹腔和骨盆腔的其餘部分。異位腎臟 (ectopic kidney) 可能位於腹腔下方或骨盆腔內，也可能位於對側；腎臟甚至可能融合

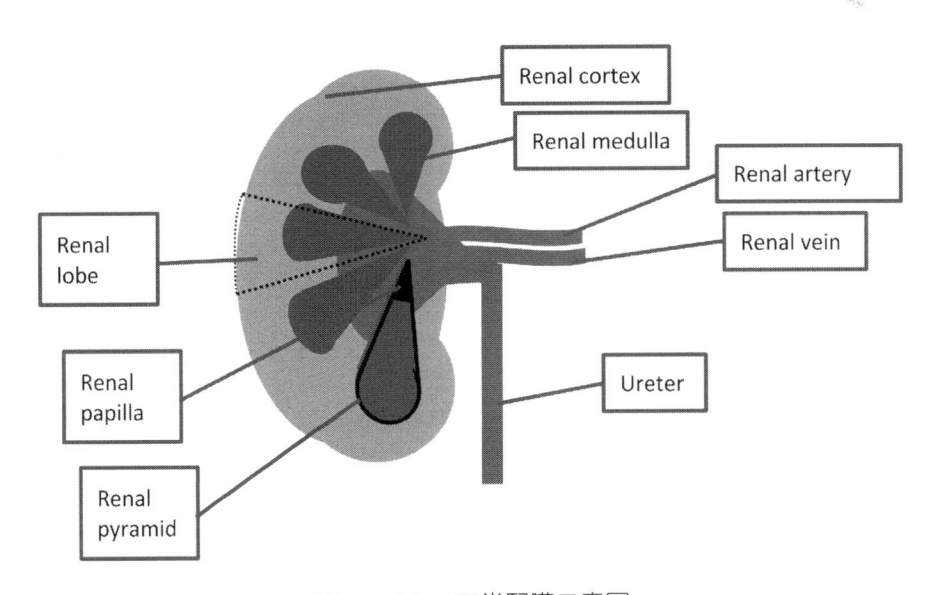

Figure 6-1. 正常腎臟示意圖

Chapter 6 Imaging: Diagnostic Characteristics of Common Kidney Diseases

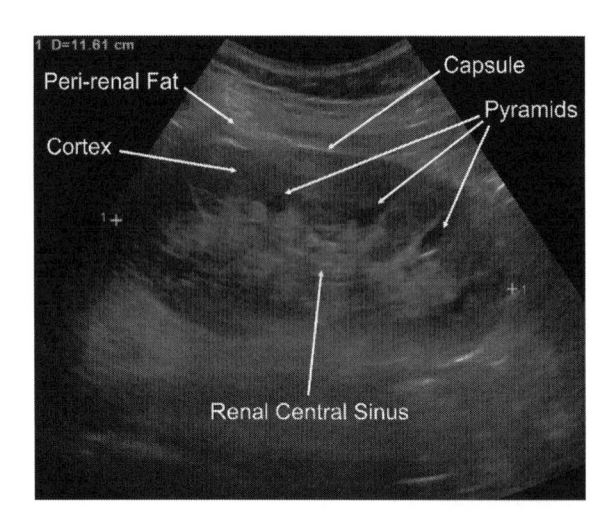

Figure 6-2. 正常腎臟超音波影像。腎臟外緣為高回音性的腎包膜 (capsule)，其內為腎實質，包括低回音性的腎錐體 (pyramid) 與中回音性的腎皮質 (cortex)。腎臟中央則為高回音性之腎竇 (renal sinus)。

（例如馬蹄腎 [horseshoe kidney]）。馬蹄腎往往位於後腹腔較低的位置，其軸可能與正常腎臟的軸不同。

超音波可以透過腎臟大小、回音性強度以及是否存在腎積水和囊性疾病來幫助區分末期腎疾病 (end-stage renal disease) 與可能可逆的急性腎損傷 (acute kidney injury) 或慢性腎實質病變 (chronic renal parenchymal disease)。腎損傷患者的腎臟周圍可能會出現回音性減弱的薄邊緣 (thin rim)，也稱為腎汗液 (renal sweat)。小的、腎實質回音性增加的腎臟則顯示病人為慢性腎病變。除了腎積水與腎動脈狹窄引起之高血壓外，很少急性可逆性腎損傷之病因可由影像學診斷。如果在超音波上未發現急性腎損傷病因，則無需進一步的影像學檢查。

（一）腎臟皮質

一般的腎臟皮質厚度約 15 mm。皮質變薄是晚期慢性腎臟病的表現。長期腎臟病變會導致腎臟萎縮，皮質變薄。皮質變厚則一般是因為水腫或發炎。與同位置的肝臟或脾臟相比，腎皮質在成人的回音性應該比肝脾來得低。如果有纖維化或細胞浸潤的話則回音性會增加 (increased echogenicity)。

在慢性腎臟病病人，腎臟超音波可以看到雙側腎臟皮質回音性增加。皮質回音增加程度與腎間質纖維化、腎小球硬化及局灶性腎小管萎縮的嚴重程度呈正相關。隨著皮質回音性增強，正常的皮質髓質分化 (corticomedullary differentiation) 喪失。然而，某些急性腎損傷患者的腎皮質回音性也可能增強，如腎小球腎炎和狼瘡性腎炎。我們可以透過連續的監測腎臟大小和皮質回音性來評估疾病的進展。

（二）腎髓質錐體

髓質的回音性比皮質低，而腎髓質疾病則會增加回音性。

（三）腎竇

在正常成人腎竇只表現 echogenic fat。超音波下集尿系統的 calyces 應該是看不見的，除非少數狀況如施打利尿劑或阻塞性腎水腫。

（四）腎囊腫的超音波影像

腎囊腫是由腎小管分化出的上皮 (epithelium) 包住液體的病灶。在超音波下可見黑色無回音性 (anechoic) 結構並有遠端回音增強 (distal enhancement)。腎囊腫可分為單純性 (simple) 與複雜性 (complex) 腎囊腫。單純性腎囊腫特徵是圓形、邊界清楚、壁光滑，和相鄰腎實質之間有清楚的界面。囊腫內液體為無回音性，可能可見薄隔膜 (septa)，但不應出現結節 (Figure 6-3)。不符合單純性腎囊腫定義則為複雜性腎囊腫，其囊腫壁較厚，合併鈣化或是囊腫內有二個以上的隔膜。複雜性腎囊腫常需以 CT 或磁振造影 (magnetic resonance imaging, MRI) 進一步檢查。

最常見的腎囊腫是偶發後天性腎囊腫 (sporadic acquired cyst)，可在正常腎臟出現。如果有許多顆囊腫則要考慮後天性囊腫腎疾病 (acquired cystic kidney disease) 或是體染色體顯性多囊腎病 (autosomal dominant polycystic kidney disease, ADPKD)。ADPKD 是常見的遺傳性多囊性腎臟疾病。超音波可以觀察到雙側腎臟增大，呈明顯分葉狀，並包含多個大小不一的無回音性區域。

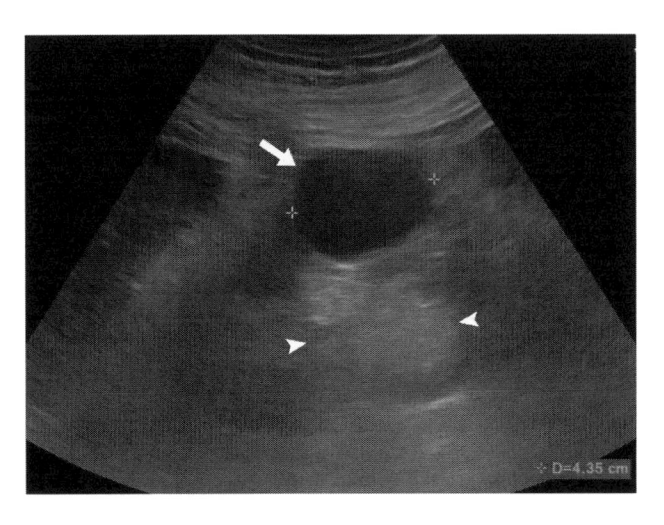

Figure 6-3. 單純性腎囊腫 (simple renal cyst) 之超音波影像。單純性腎囊腫之超音波影像為薄壁、無回音性的圓型構造（箭號），並具有遠端回音增強 (distal enhancement) 現象（箭頭）。

（五）泌尿道阻塞 (Urinary Obstruction) 的超音波影像

泌尿道阻塞一般會導致腎積水 (hydronephrosis)，其代表集尿系統擴大，特別是小腎盞與大腎盞。一般而言，腎積水會使腎臟的長度和整體尺寸變大。在急性泌尿道阻塞期，腎臟皮質會是完整的，然而慢性泌尿道阻塞可能導致腎實質萎縮，腎臟尺寸變小與腎皮質變薄。腎積水在超音波影像的表現為擴張而充滿液體的腎盂和腎盞 (Figure 6-4)。根據腎盞擴張程度和皮質變薄程度可將腎積水分成四級：

1. 輕度（I 級）腎積水

腎盂腎盞系統 (pelvicalyceal system) 充滿液體，導致中央腎竇脂肪輕微分離。腎盞不變形，腎皮質厚度正常。

2. 中度（II 級）腎積水

腎盂腎盞系統更加膨脹，中央腎竇分離程度更大。腎盞的輪廓變成圓形，但皮質厚度沒有改變。

3. 中度至重度（III 級）腎積水

腎盞更加膨脹，並且可以看到皮質變薄。

4. 嚴重（IV 級）腎積水

腎盞系統明顯擴張。腎盞表現為大的、氣球狀的、充滿液體的結構，具有大小不一擴張的腎盂。擴張的腎盞接近或到達腎包膜。

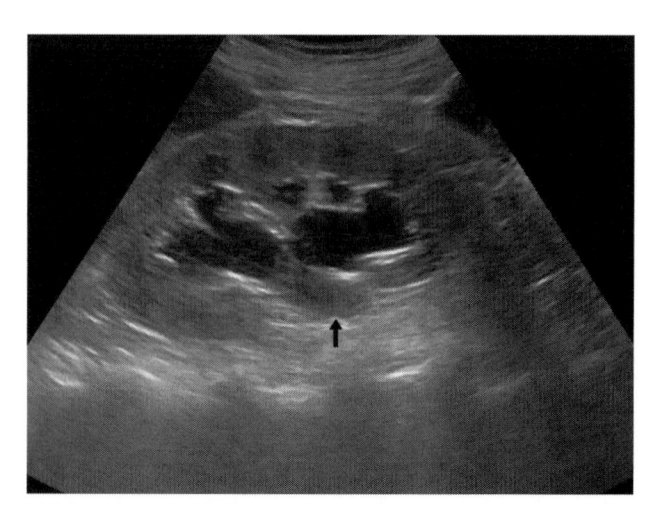

Figure 6-4. 腎積水 (hydronephrosis) 之超音波影像。典型腎積水影像，可見擴大的腎盞 (calyx)、腎盂 (pelvis) 和輸尿管（ureter，見箭號指向處）。

然腎積水通常很容易透過超音波診斷，但需要和囊性腎臟疾病作鑑別診斷。在腎積水中，擴張的腎盞與腎盂有明顯的直接聯繫，腎盂也是擴張的。而在囊性腎臟疾病中。充滿液體的圓形囊腫有壁，每個腎盞和腎盂之間沒有明顯的直接聯繫。腎盂周圍囊腫 (parapelvic cyst) 病例經常被誤診為腎盂擴張。腎動脈瘤也可能與擴張的腎盂混淆，但可以藉著都卜勒彩色血流超音波來正確診斷。

（六）腎臟結石 (Renal Stone) 與鈣化 (Calcification) 的超音波影像

超音波是檢查腎結石很有用的檢查，可能可以觀察到合併有單側腎臟積水。腎結石會反射幾乎全部的音波，因此是產生回音性的白亮色病灶，並有遠端陰影 (distal shadow) (Figure 6-5)。不論結石組成成份為何，在超音波下的表現皆相同。由於超音波受到腸氣阻擋，輸尿管的結石很少可以看到。若結石位於輸尿管膀胱交界 (ureterovesical junction, UVJ) 處的遠端輸尿管則可從充滿尿液的膀胱觀察。超音波可以顯示結石通過一側的膀胱中沒有輸尿管射流 (jet)。

（七）腫瘤 (Neoplasm) 的超音波影像

1. 腎細胞癌 (Renal Cell Carcinoma, RCC) 與泌尿道上皮癌 (Urothelial Cell Carcinoma)

RCC 在超音波下的典型表現是界線清楚的低回音性腫塊，並會使腎臟輪廓扭曲 (Figure 6-6)。但是當 RCC 小於 3 cm 時，有可能呈現等回音性 (isoechoic) 或高回音性。有 10% RCC 看起來像腎囊腫。

泌尿道上皮癌於腎臟則是源自腎盂的腫瘤，典型表現是在腎盂內的低回音性腫塊，並藉由脂肪組織和腎實質隔開。

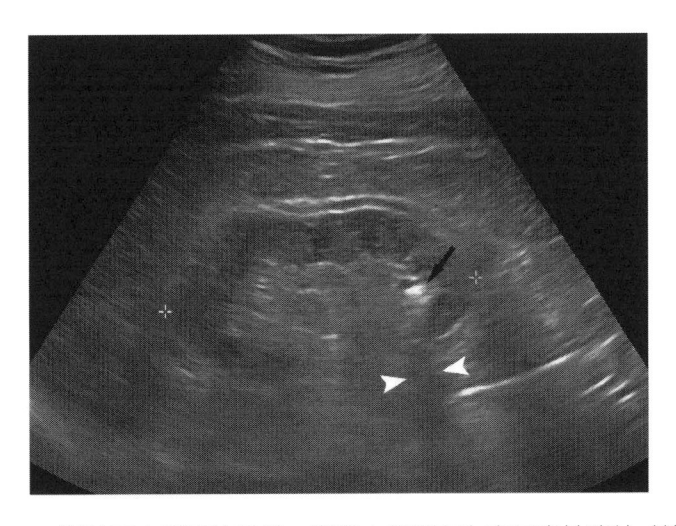

Figure 6-5. 腎結石之超音波影像。腎盞之腎結石為高回音性病灶（箭號），並有黑色遠端聲音陰影（箭頭）。

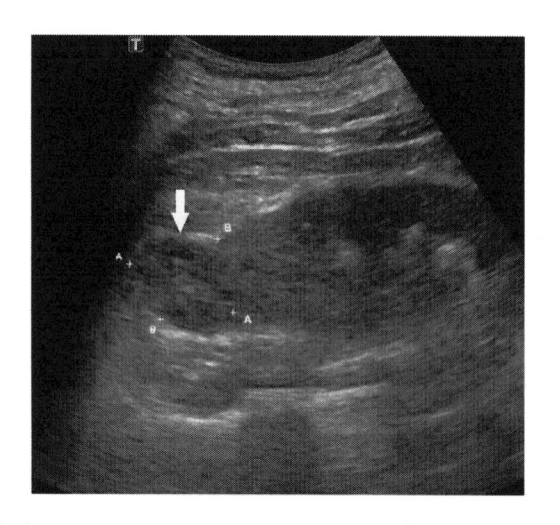

Figure 6-6. 腎細胞癌 (renal cell carcinoma, RCC) 之超音波影像。在腎臟上極 (upper pole) 處有一界線清楚的低回音腫塊（箭頭），但在其後沒有遠端回音增強 (enhancement)，可和腎囊腫鑑別。此圖為 RCC 的典型超音波表現。

2. 血管肌肉脂肪瘤 (Angiomyolipoma, AML)

AML 是成人最常見的良性腎臟腫瘤。是由不同組織組成的良性腎腫瘤，包括血管、肌肉、脂肪等成分，亦可能包含軟骨組織。超音波典型表現是亮白色高回音性腫瘤，歸因於腫瘤內高比例的脂肪成份，但和結石或鈣化不同處是沒有遠端聲音陰影 (acoustic shadow) (Figure 6-7)。

二、CT

腎臟在無顯影 CT 掃描影像為軟組織密度 (soft tissue density) 之卵圓形構造，並被脂肪包圍。脂肪密度為 –30 亨氏單位 (Hounsfield unit, HU) 或更低，所以呈暗黑色，而脂肪在打顯影劑後會變亮。鈣化、骨頭以及含碘顯影劑 (iodinated contrast) 之密度一般則大於 100 HU，呈現亮白色。腎功能不好的病人使用含碘顯影劑會有急性腎損傷風險，但由於 CT 相較於 MRI，不僅便宜也較快速，因此在腎臟疾病的評估比 MRI 來的普遍。一般 CT 可由以下幾個期相 (phase) 以判別腎臟病灶 (Figure 6-8)：

（一）無顯影相 (non-contrast phase)：可評估腎結石、高密度囊腫和輪廓異常。

（二）早期動脈相 (early arterial phase)：顯影劑靜脈注射 12–15 秒後之影像，當顯影劑到達腎動脈 (renal artery) 時開始，而在顯影劑腎臟靜脈回流 (renal venous return) 前結束。此期相可瞭解腎動脈解剖構造與診斷血管病變（如腎動脈狹窄），但對腎臟或泌尿道的病灶影像診斷幫助不大。

腎臟醫學臨床技能手冊 第二版

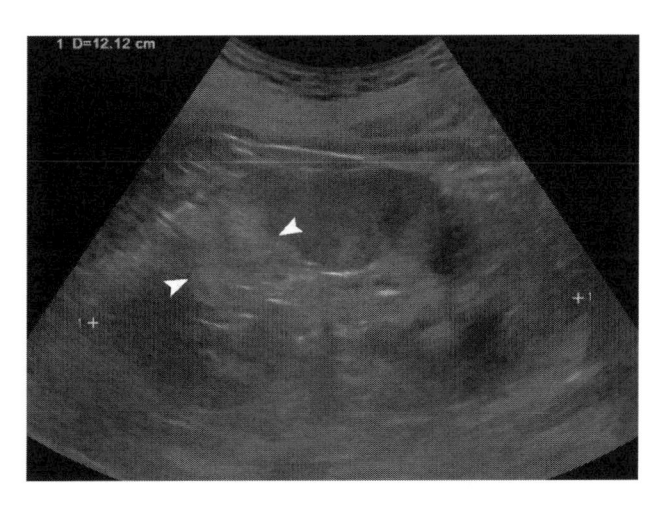

Figure 6-7. 血管肌肉脂肪瘤 (angiomyolipoma) 之超音波影像。腎臟實質中有一亮白產生回音性 (echogenic) 病灶,但缺乏遠端陰影 (distal shadowing),因此可和腎結石作區分。

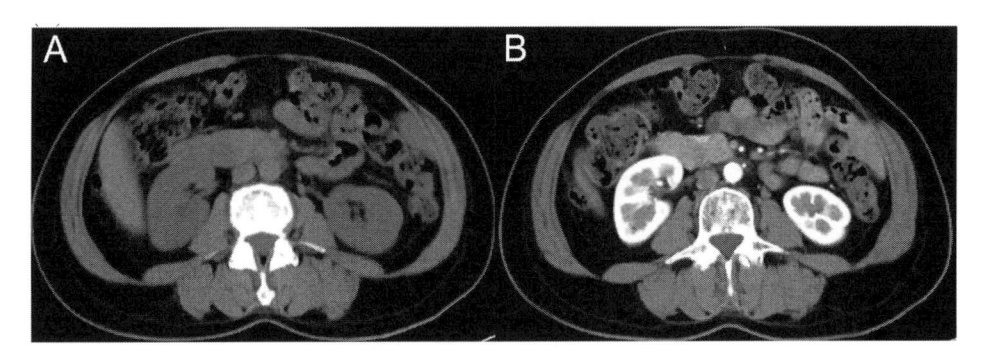

Figure 6-8. 正常腎臟之電腦斷層 (computed tomography) 影像。(A) 無顯影相 (non-contrast phase)。(B) 皮質髓質相 (corticomedullary phase)。

（三）皮質髓質相 (corticomedullary phase)：顯影劑靜脈注射 25–30 秒後之影像,以皮質顯影為主,結束在顯影劑產生腎髓質顯影之前,用於腎臟腫瘤的評估。正常的腎皮質與高血管性 (hypervascular) 腫塊在此期相會呈現高度顯影增強。

（四）腎臟造影相 (nephrographic phase)：顯影劑靜脈注射 90–100 秒後整個腎實質會呈現均勻顯影,皮質髓質分化無法出現。此期相最容易偵測在皮質或髓質的病灶。

（五）延遲／排出相 (delayed/excretory phase)：約在注射顯影劑後 3 分鐘開始攝影,此時集尿系統因顯影劑排出而呈現高亮度,若有集尿系統的微小病灶會呈現為顯影缺陷 (filling defect)。可以評估集尿系統構造（腎盞、腎盂、輸尿管和膀胱）。

Chapter 6 Imaging: Diagnostic Characteristics of Common Kidney Diseases

（一）泌尿道阻塞的 CT 影像

　　CT 影像可見擴張且充滿液體之腎臟集尿系統與輸尿管。急性阻塞的腎臟會水腫變大。由於顯影劑排出受阻，因此皮質髓質相時間延長，變成持續性腎臟造影，而顯影劑排至集尿系統的時間亦隨之延遲 (Figure 6-9)。慢性阻塞會造成明顯擴張且充滿液體之集尿系統和萎縮之腎實質 (Figure 6-10)。

（二）腎臟結石與鈣化的 CT 影像

　　腹部 CT 對腎臟結石的敏感性為 96% 至 100%，特異性為 95% 至 100%，準確率為 96% 至 98%。而靜脈腎盂造影 (intravenous pyelography, IVP) 的敏感性為 64% 至

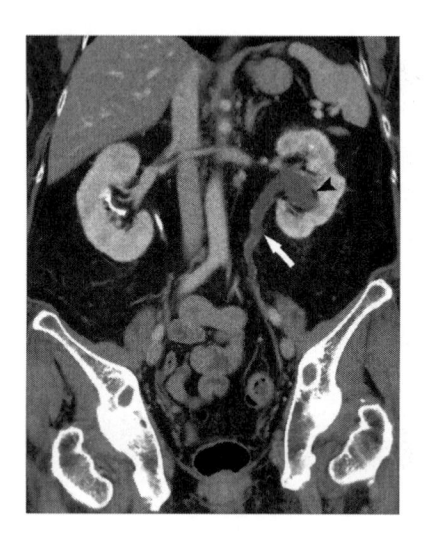

Figure 6-9. 腎積水 (hydronephrosis) 之電腦斷層 (computed tomography, CT) 影像。此為腎積水的典型 CT 影像。阻塞處是左側腎臟（箭頭），可見擴張之腎盂與輸尿管，充滿低密度的尿液。

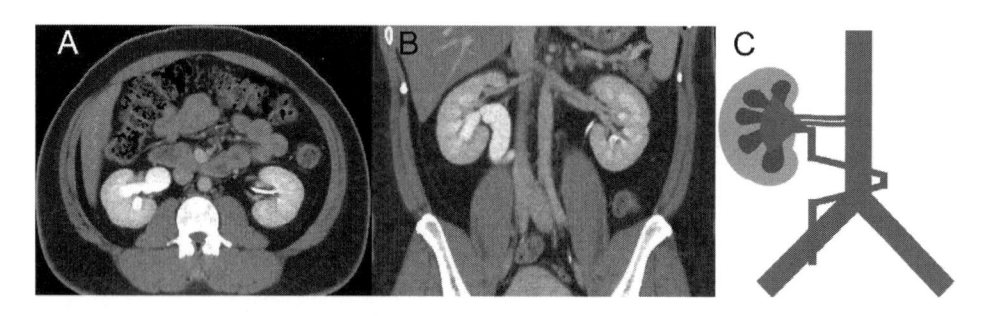

Figure 6-10. 下腔靜脈後輸尿管 (retrocaval ureter) 造成腎積水之電腦斷層 (computed tomography) 影像。下腔靜脈後輸尿管造成右腎積水，可看到擴大的腎盂和輸尿管（A, B）。下腔靜脈後輸尿管之示意圖（C）。

97%，特異性為 92% 至 94%。超音波的敏感性為則為 24%，特異性為 90%。因此 CT 掃描已經成為檢測腎結石最常使用的工具。在懷疑腎結石的病人，應該先安排無顯影 CT 掃描檢查，因為顯影劑排出至集尿系統會遮蔽潛在的鈣化或結石。最常見的結石阻塞位置是在三處解剖狹窄處：輸尿管腎盂交界處 (ureteropelvic junction)、輸尿管跨過總髂動脈 (common iliac artery) 或外髂動脈 (external iliac artery) 處，即骨盆緣 (pelvic brim) 以及 UVJ。腎結石 CT 影像之典型表現是高密度亮白色病灶（其亮度視結石成分而定，但皆比軟組織亮）(Figure 6-11)，亦可能伴隨阻塞側的輸尿管擴張、腎周圍脂肪 (perinephric fat) 浸潤、腎積水及腎臟腫大等變化。

（三）腎囊腫與腎腫塊 (mass) 的 CT 影像

腎囊腫之典型 CT 影像為邊界清楚的圓形水密度病灶，壁很薄，注射顯影劑後密度不增加。囊腫內液體含量可能和水的密度略有不同，但原則上不超過 10–5 HU。腎囊腫與相鄰腎實質的交界面清晰且邊緣光滑，沒有明顯的結節，但可能可見薄層鈣化。有時可遇到密度為 50–80 HU 的「高密度」腎囊腫，這些多是出血或含有高蛋白質成分的囊腫。與單純性囊腫一樣，它們應該沒有壁結節，並且注射顯影劑後密度沒有明顯增強。高密度囊腫常見於多囊腎。

西元 1986 年，學者 Bosniak 依據 CT 影像將腎囊腫分類，之後陸續在 2012 年與 2019 年作過修改。目前最新的版本是將腎囊腫根據影像表現（包括 CT 與 MRI）分成以下幾類：

1. Type I：簡單的良性囊腫 (benign simple cyst)，不須追蹤。
2. Type II：良性，有薄間隔 (≤ 2 mm) 的囊腫。
3. Type IIF：水泡性囊腫有平滑而稍微增厚 (3 mm) 的壁或隔間，或是多個 (≥ 4) 平滑而薄 (≤ 2 mm) 的隔間。
4. Type III：水泡性囊腫有不平滑或增厚 (≥ 4 mm) 的壁或隔間。

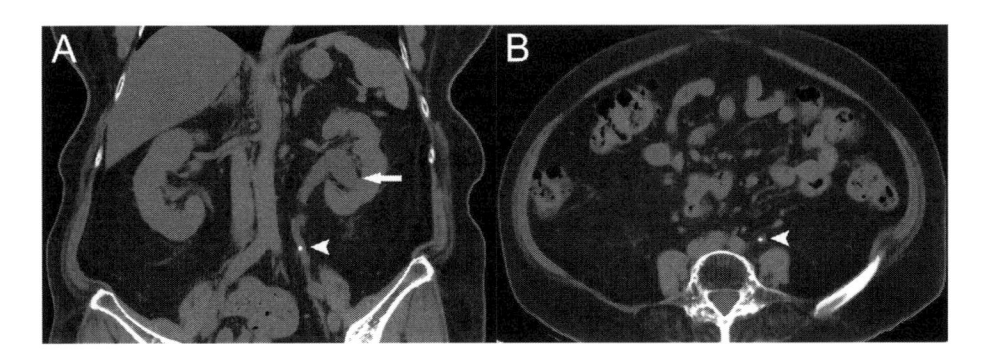

Figure 6-11. 腎結石之電腦斷層 (computed tomography, CT) 影像。典型腎結石的無顯影 CT 影像，可見擴張的腎盂（A: 箭號）與亮白色輸尿管結石（A, B: 箭頭）。

5. Type IV：明顯惡性，在囊腫壁上有軟組織密度或可顯影結節 (enhancing nodule)。

ADPKD 之 CT 影像為擴大的分葉狀腎臟合併大小不一的囊腫，囊腫壁可能有鈣化。由於囊腫常常合併出血，因此常有密度或亮度不同的囊腫。此外在肝臟、脾臟和胰臟中也可能發現囊腫 (Figure 6-12)。

（四）AML 之 CT 影像

AML 因為含有大量脂肪，CT 影像會顯示出 low attenuation (< −10 HU)。

（五）RCC 之 CT 影像

RCC 的 CT 影像為邊緣不規則之腫塊或結節，未打顯影劑時其密度可能接近腎實質 (isoattenuating)，亦可能較腎實質低 (hypoattenuating) 或高 (hyperattenuating)。但注射顯影劑後，RCC 會顯影，特別是在腎臟造影相更明顯。而在皮質髓質相則可釐清腫瘤和血管構造的關聯。透明細胞 (clear cell) 型 RCC 通常比乳突 (papillary) 型顯得更不均質 (Figure 6-13)。而嫌色 (chromophobe) 型通常表現為均質。乳突型和嫌色型 RCC 常常合併鈣化點。RCC 中間也可能出現低密度壞死區域。有時 RCC 也以囊腫性腫塊 (cystic mass) 表現，合併囊腫內厚間隔 (thick septa) 與囊腫壁結節 (wall nodularity)。

（六）黃色肉芽腫性腎盂腎炎 (Xanthogranulomatous Pyelonephritis, XPN) 之 CT 影像

XPN 是一少見慢性腎盂腎炎 (chronic pyelonephritis) 之變型 (variant)。常導因於感染性腎結石造成集尿系統阻塞之慢性發炎疾病，腎實質與腎周圍脂肪被含脂肪 (lipid-laden) 巨噬細胞之肉芽腫性組織所取代。CT 影像特徵為腎實質被許多邊緣顯影之圓型

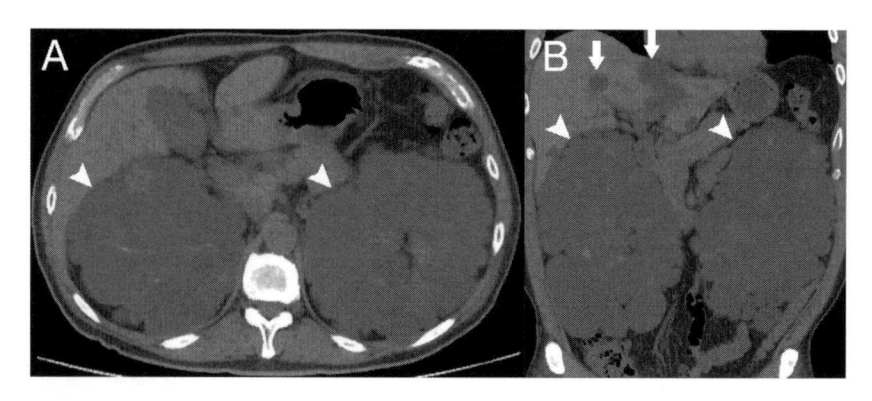

Figure 6-12. 多囊腎病之顯影增強 (contrast-enhanced) 電腦斷層 (computed tomography) 影像，雙側腎臟充滿大小不一圓型囊腫（A, B: 箭頭），其密度未受顯影劑增強，較肝臟與主動脈為低。亦可於肝臟發現許多囊腫（B: 箭號）。

低密度 (15-18 HU) 區域所取代，產生多囊室性 (multiloculated) 外觀。因該影像類似熊掌，故名為熊掌徵象 (bear paw sign) (Figure 6-14)。

三、MRI

MRI 成像原理為當病人位於產生靜磁場電磁鐵之中心孔 (central bore) 時，人體細胞中含有總數為奇數之質子或中子的原子核（主要為水分子的氫原子核）會產生磁力向量（磁矩），此磁矩方向會與靜磁場方向平行 (parallel) 或反平行（antiparallel，Z 軸分量）。當施加與氫原子核旋進 (precession) 頻率相同，但與磁矩方向呈 90 度角的射頻脈衝 (radiofrequency pulse) 後，可使這些氫原子核從低能量狀態變成高能量狀態（激發，excitation），且將磁矩從縱向（Z 軸方向）偏轉至橫向（X-Y 軸方向），使其淨磁矩變成垂直主磁場方向。當射頻脈衝停止後，氫原子核會從高能量狀態回到平衡狀態（弛緩，relaxation），所釋放之能量會轉為射頻訊號，並被接收轉換成影

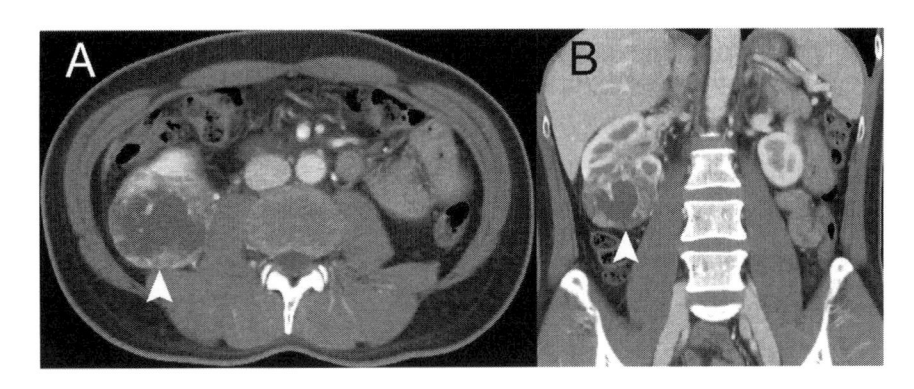

Figure 6-13. 腎細胞癌 (renal cell carcinoma, RCC) 之電腦斷層 (computed tomography) 影像。注射顯影劑後，RCC 為可顯影，邊緣不規則腫塊。此案例合併有低密度腫瘤中心壞死區域（箭頭）。

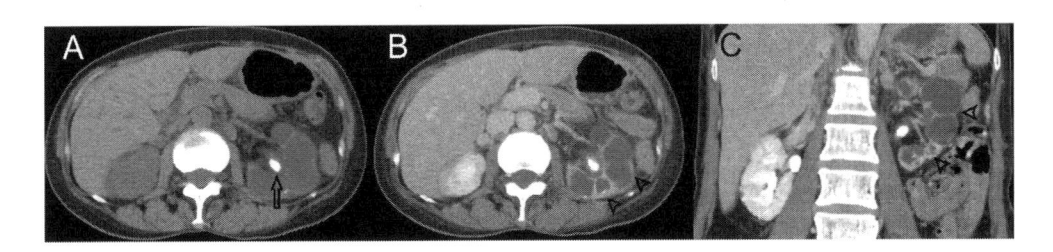

Figure 6-14. 黃色肉芽腫性腎盂腎炎 (xanthogranulomatous pyelonephritis, XPN) 之電腦斷層 (computed tomography, CT) 影像。XPN 的無顯影 CT 影像可見高密度腎結石（A: 箭號）。顯影劑注射後可見腎盂區域壞死併擴張，合併邊緣顯影，呈現熊掌徵象 (bear paw sign)（B, C: 箭頭）。

像。弛緩過程分成兩個過程，分別是 Z 軸分量的回復與 X-Y 軸分量的歸零。射頻脈衝停止後，氫原子核將所獲得的能量以熱能方式傳遞到周圍組織，使 Z 軸分量回復到基態 63% 所需時間，稱為 T1 弛緩時間 (T1 relaxation time)，又稱為自旋－晶格弛緩時間 (spin-lattice relaxation time)；X-Y 軸分量衰減 63% 所需時間則稱為 T2 弛緩時間 (T2 relaxation time)，又稱為自旋－自旋弛緩時間 (spin-spin relaxation time)。重複兩次射頻脈衝之間的時間稱為重複時間 (repetition time, TR)，決定多少 Z 軸分量可回復 (T1 relaxation)。產生射頻脈衝至感應線圈接收到氫原子核能量釋放轉成之射頻訊號之間的時間稱為回音時間 (echo time, TE)，決定多少 X-Y 軸分量可回復 (T2 relaxation)，TE 常小於 TR。利用人體各組織與體液之質子含量、T1 弛緩時間、T2 弛緩時間不同，便可分辨各組織之磁振影像。例如每單位體積之尿液所含質子較腎組織為多，但腎結石所含之質子便遠少於腎組織。影像之信號強度 (signal intensity) 與所接收到回傳之組織射頻訊號成正比，而組織射頻訊號與該次射頻脈衝後剩餘的橫向磁矩分量 (M_{XY}) 及下次射頻脈衝前所回復之縱向磁矩分量 (M_Z) 呈正相關。

　　一般而言，磁振影像可分為 T1 加權影像 (T1-weighted image) 與 T2 加權影像 (T2-weighted image)。T1 加權影像所設定之 TR（常 < 500 毫秒 [ms]）與 TE（常 < 30 ms）均較短，可凸顯組織間 T1 弛緩時間之差異；T1 加權影像中，T1 弛緩時間短的組織（如脂肪、新鮮出血）有較多的縱向 Z 軸分量回復 (M_Z)，因此信號強度較高，呈現白色。反之 T1 弛緩時間長的組織（如腫瘤、水腫、發炎、腦脊液、體液等）信號強度較低，呈現暗黑色。T2 加權影像所設定之 TR（常 > 1,500 ms）與 TE（常 > 90 ms）均較長，一般而言為 T1 加權影像設定值 3 倍以上，可凸顯組織間 T2 弛緩時間之差異；T2 加權影像中，T2 弛緩時間長的組織（如水腫、發炎、腦脊液、體液、神經膠狀變性 [gliosis] 等），M_{XY} 衰減較慢，有較多的剩餘 M_{XY}，故呈現亮白色高信號強度。正常肝臟之 T2 弛緩時間較短，故呈現暗黑色。

　　MRI 雖較少用於鑑別腎臟病變，但在需區分腎臟病灶的種類或腎臟周邊組織時，仍有一定角色。在 T1 加權影像，腎臟會呈現灰色，如同腹腔臟器和肌肉；於 T2 加權影像中，腎臟信號強度略高，如同脾臟一般。腎髓質在 T1 加權影像會比腎皮質暗，但在 T2 加權影像比腎皮質亮，這可能是因為腎髓質含較多性質屬自由流動水份 (unbound water) 之尿液。而腎盞、腎盂和輸尿管則因為富含尿液，因此在 T1 加權影像是暗黑色，但在 T2 加權影像是亮白色。腎周脂肪 (perirenal fat) 則在 T1 與 T2 加權影像均呈亮白色，故常利用影像抑制技術將此亮白色脂肪影像消除，以利辨別含脂肪之腎臟病灶，如 AML (Figure 6-15)。而血管影像之亮度則不一定，根據脈衝序列 (pulse sequence)、成像平面與是否使用含釓 (gadolinium) 顯影劑而有所不同。在腎絲球過濾率 (glomerular filtration rate) 每分鐘小於 30 mL 的病人使用含釓顯影劑有引起腎因性全身纖維化 (nephrogenic systemic fibrosis) 的風險，不得不慎。

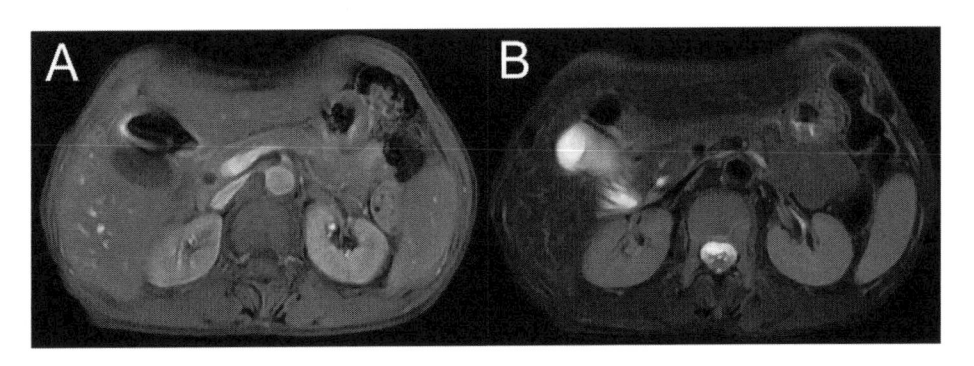

Figure 6-15. 正常腎臟之磁振造影 (magnetic resonance imaging, MRI) 影像。典型的正常腎臟 MRI 影像。(A) 經顯影劑注射後之 T1 加權影像併有脂肪抑制，可見到主動脈呈亮白色，膽囊與脊椎中之腦脊液為暗黑色。(B) T1 加權影像併有脂肪抑制，可見到膽囊與腦脊液為亮白色，腎組織灰度與脾臟相近，腎髓質較腎皮質亮。

（一）泌尿道阻塞的 MRI 影像

MRI 並非泌尿道阻塞的第一線影像檢查，但在不適用 CT 病人（如對含碘顯影劑過敏者）仍可使用，且不見得需要使用含釓顯影劑才能辨別阻塞處。

泌尿道結石在 T1 和 T2 加權影像中都呈暗黑色，因此結石在擴張的集尿系統中十分明顯。急性泌尿道阻塞可在 T2 加權影像觀察到腎臟周圍的積液。而在腎結石術後的病人，MRI 對於區分腎內和腎外的血腫比 CT 更加準確。

（二）腎臟結石與鈣化的 MRI 影像

腎臟或輸尿管鈣化在 MRI 上因無訊號故不可見。在磁振影像上可能會以黑色無訊號的局部病灶表現。但空氣、金屬或縫線也會有同樣的表現。

（三）腎囊腫的 MRI 影像

由於 MRI 可清楚分辨軟組織的對比度，因此對於囊腫的顯示可以非常明顯。腎囊腫在 T1 加權影像為暗黑色，在 T2 加權影像則是亮白色。複雜的囊腫含有蛋白質或出血性液體，可能有分隔和鈣化。

四、核子醫學影像 (Nuclear Medicine Image)：腎圖 (Renography)

腎圖是最常使用的核醫腎臟學檢查。其作用原理是放射示蹤劑 (radiotracer) 經靜脈注射後，隨血流進入腎臟，由腎小管上皮細胞吸收後分泌到腎小管腔內，再隨尿液匯集到腎盂，最終由輸尿管排入膀胱。用腎圖儀的兩個放射性探測器或加瑪照

相機在體表分別記錄兩腎臟區域之時間 - 放射性曲線，透過比較兩側腎臟，可知是否有單側腎功能異常或尿路是否通暢 (Figure 6-16)。目前最常用的示蹤劑是 ^{131}I- 鄰碘馬尿酸 (^{131}I-ortho-iodo-hippurate) 及鎝-99m 巰基乙醯三甘氨酸 (technetium-99m-mercaptoacetyltriglycine)。本檢查的主要優點是能夠提供單側腎功能和單側上段尿路通暢情況，並且操作簡便價廉、無痛苦創傷且安全，對體弱者、小兒和含碘顯影劑過敏者也適用。主要的缺點是圖形缺乏特異性，難以單純根據圖形作出疾病診斷。此外，技術性因素較多，不加注意會影響結果的精確性。但密切結合其他臨床資訊可發揮很大診斷價值。Table 1 為不同腎圖檢查適應症：

五、IVP

IVP 是用來檢查泌尿系統（含腎臟、輸尿管與膀胱）有無異常的特殊 X 光檢查。經靜脈注射含碘顯影劑後，血中之顯影劑由腎臟排至腎盂，再經由輸尿管進入膀胱。透過在特定時間點照射腹部 X 光，觀察顯影劑的流動與顯影，可顯示泌尿系統的結構

Table 1. 各式腎圖檢查與適應症

腎圖檢查與適應症
Basic renogram
評估腎功能和尿路動力學
確定每顆腎臟貢獻多少比例的總體腎功能
Diuresis renogram
診斷或排除尿路阻塞
ACE inhibition (RVH or captopril renogram)
診斷或排除 RVH
Renal transplant scintigraphy
評估動脈血流量和功能
幫助診斷移植腎排斥和急性腎小管壞死
診斷 urinary leak, infarct, 或 outflow obstruction
Renal cortical scintigraphy
診斷或排除腎盂腎炎
確定每顆腎臟貢獻多少比例的總體腎功能
Radionuclide cystography
診斷、定量和監測尿液逆流 (reflux)
評估有尿液逆流的小孩的無症狀兄弟姊妹

Abbreviations: ACE, angiotensin-converting enzyme; RVH, renovascular hypertension.

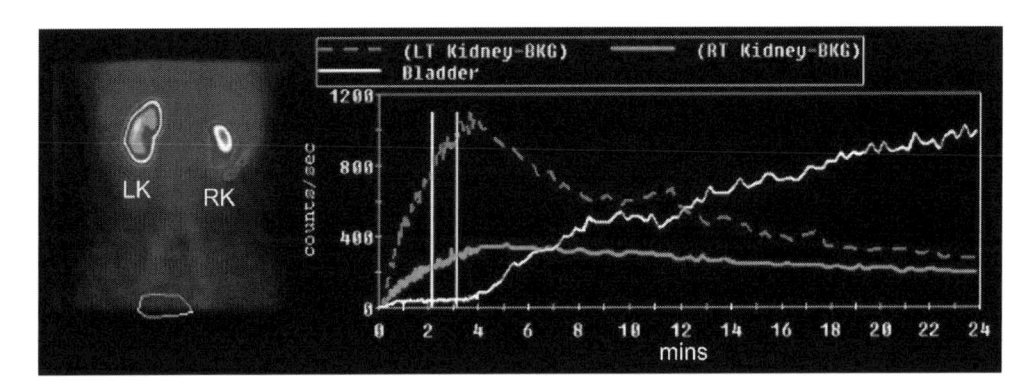

Figure 6-16. 腎功能異常之核子醫學腎圖影像。一位右腎功能不良病患的 ^{99m}Tc-MAG3 檢查結果。由核醫檢查結果可發現此病人的右腎 (right kidney, RK) 功能大幅減少；同時腎圖顯示左腎 (left kidney, LK) 尿液排出圖形有波動，暗示可能有尿液逆流。

與是否有結石、腫瘤、尿路阻塞或各種泌尿道畸形。因需注射含碘顯影劑，故需注意病人是否有含碘顯影劑過敏、腎功能異常或甲狀腺疾病史。

典型的 IVP 步驟如下：

（一）請患者先平躺，照第一張腹部 X 光片 (kidney, ureter, bladder [KUB])。此 X 光片為顯影前，可以觀察病患原本的構造包含脊椎、骨盆、大腸、小腸等。

（二）注射顯影劑 5 分鐘後照相。此時可能會使用束腹帶壓迫腹部使腎臟顯影劑較佳。這組 X 光片可以觀察到雙側腎臟開始顯影，亦可比較雙側腎臟顯影速度，腎功能不佳之腎臟其顯影劑排泄速度會變慢，甚至無法顯影。

（三）注射顯影劑 10–15 分鐘後照相。此時會將束腹帶解開，讓顯影劑往下自然流動，再照 X 光。此時可觀察顯影劑於輸尿管內流動的情況，並可比較雙側輸尿管是否有阻塞或結構異常。

（四）注射顯影劑 30 分鐘後照相。此時可以在膀胱觀察到顯影劑顯影，若膀胱壁呈不規則形狀或有顯影劑充盈缺損，則可能有膀胱腫瘤。

（五）注射顯影劑 60 分鐘與排尿後 (post-voiding) 會再照一張可以觀察膀胱排尿後的情況。可依據顯影劑流動的情況與病人病情加照 X 光。

IVP 之應用情形眾多，藉比較兩側腎臟顯影的速度，可初步判別個別腎臟之功能是否異常。腎功能不佳之腎臟其顯影劑排泄速度會變慢，甚至無法顯影。泌尿系統若有輸尿管阻塞、腎水腫 (Figure 6-17) 或畸形，大多能顯現出來。IVP 亦可偵測腎乳頭壞死 (renal papilla necrosis) 與膀胱腫瘤。藉由比較仰臥與站立 IVP 影像，若腎臟位移超過 5 cm 或 2 個椎體高度，則可診斷游離腎 (floating kidney)。然而 IVP 也有其缺點和限制，腎功能太差者無法將顯影劑排出，以致患側腎臟無法顯影；對顯影劑過敏者不能使用；有甲狀腺病史者亦需注意。

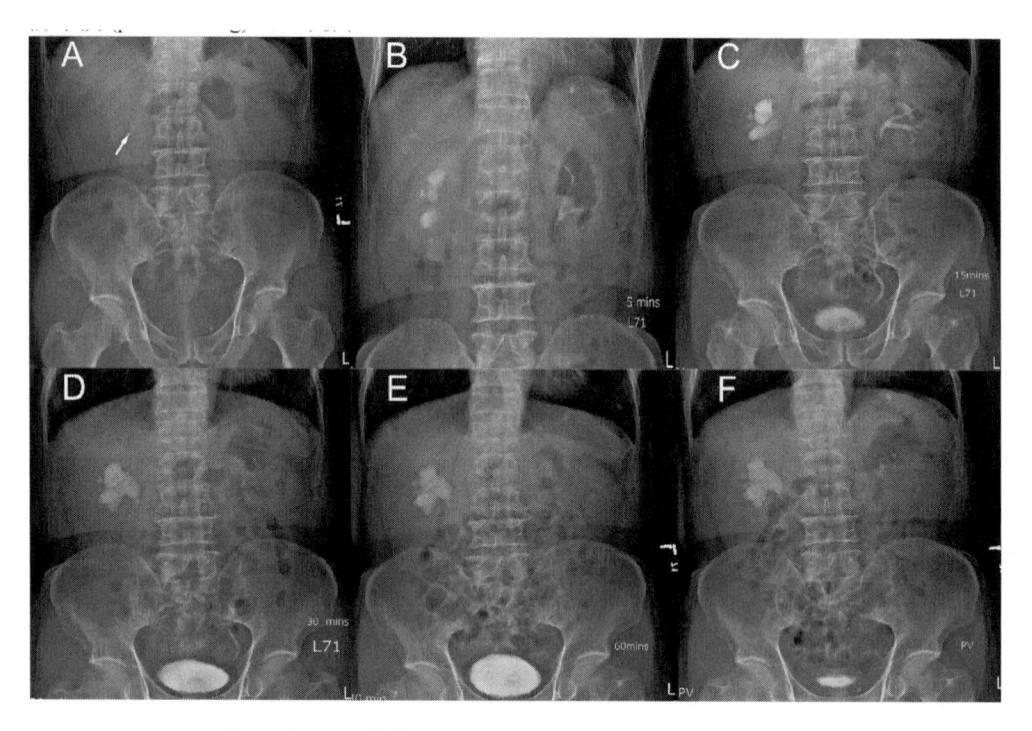

Figure 6-17. 右側輸尿管結石併腎積水之的靜脈腎盂造影 (intravenous pyelography)。(A) 注射顯影劑前的 KUB (kidney, ureter, bladder) 素片，在右側腎盂輸尿管交界處有一放射不透光性 (radiopaque) 之輸尿管結石（箭號）。(B) 至 (E) 依序為注射顯影劑後 5 分鐘、15 分鐘、30 分鐘與 60 分鐘之 X 光片，可見右側腎積水，且右側腎臟顯影劑延遲排出。(F) 為排尿後 (post-voiding) 之 X 光片。

六、KUB

　　腹部 X 光片造影檢查對於評估腎臟、輸尿管和膀胱能提供的資訊相對有限。腎臟位於上腹部後腹腔，被脂肪包圍，常常會被腸氣擋住。若在 X 光片上看到腎臟區域的鈣化點，有可能是結石（需出現在泌尿系統的路徑上），但亦可能是腎腫瘤鈣化、腎血管鈣化或其他腎組織鈣化，需要其他影像進一步協助。腎臟結石可分為 nephrolithiasis 與 nephrocalcinosis，前者之結石位於集尿系統（腎盂）；後者之結石或鈣化位於腎實質 (Figure 6-18)。腹部 X 光片僅能顯示放射不透光性 (radiopaque) 結石，如磷酸鈣、草酸鈣結石。鳥糞石 (struvite) 結石之成份為磷酸銨鎂，通常為放射不透光性，但亦有例外。放射透光性 (radiolucent) 結石則有尿酸、胱胺酸 (cystine) 與 indinavir 結石。因檢測泌尿道結石之敏感度低，故腹部 X 光片未顯示結石並無法排除此診斷。

此外腹膜透析病患可藉由 KUB 確認腹膜透析管位於在正確的位置（在 Cul-de-sac，tip 朝下）(Figure 6-19)。除此之外，包囊性腹膜硬化症 (encapsulating peritoneal sclerosis) 也可用 KUB 作第一線檢查，嚴重者可見到腸壁鈣化 (Figure 6-20)。

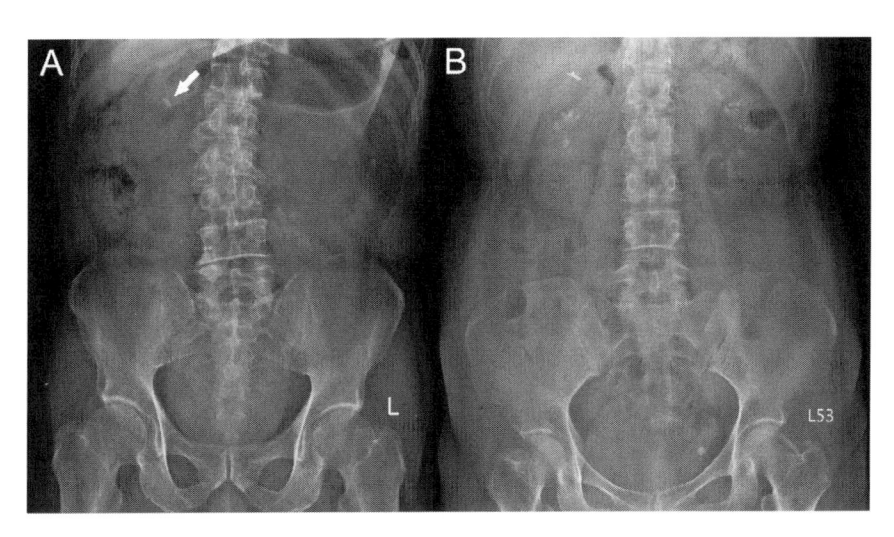

Figure 6-18. 腎臟結石的 KUB (kidney, ureter, bladder) 影像。(A) 右上腹腎臟區域可看到放射不透光之腎結石（nephrolithiasis，箭號）。(B) 則可在腎髓質看到許多鈣化點 (nephrocalcinosis)。

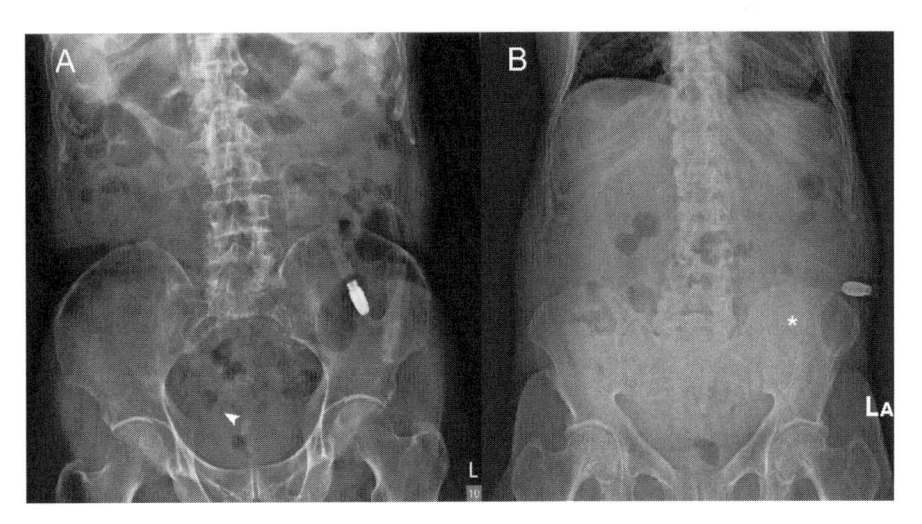

Figure 6-19. 顯示腹膜透析導管位置的 KUB (kidney, ureter, bladder)。(A) 顯示導管尖端正常朝下，位於骨盆腔低處（箭頭）。(B) 顯示導管位移 (catheter migration)，尖端朝上（星號）。

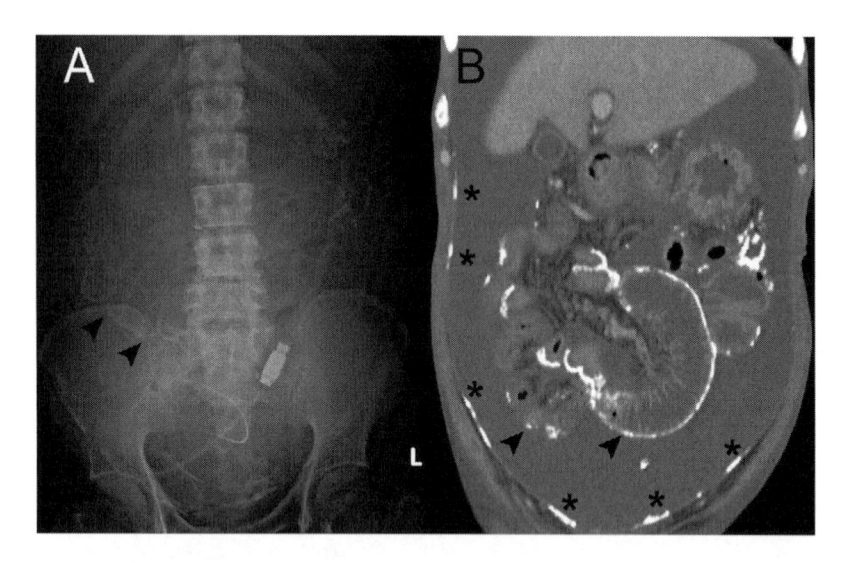

Figure 6-20. 包囊性腹膜硬化症病之 KUB (kidney, ureter, bladder) 和電腦斷層 (computed tomography, CT) 影像。(A) 是 KUB 影像，可見腸子阻塞聚集於中央，併有腸壁鈣化（箭頭）。(B) 為 CT 影像，可見腸壁鈣化（箭頭）和腹膜鈣化（星號）。

延伸閱讀文獻

Rahbari-Oskoui F, Taylor AT, O'Neill WC. Chapter 10. Ultrasonography and nuclear medicine. In: Schrier RW, Coffman TM, Falk RJ, Molitoris BA, Neilson EG, eds. *Schrier's Diseases of the Kidney*. 9th ed. Philadelphia, PA: Lippincott Williams and Wilkins; 2013:346-400.

Duddalwar VA, Jadvar H, Palmer SL. Chapter 25. Diagnostic kidney imaging. In: Skorecki K, Chertow GM, Marsden PA, Taal MW, Yu ASL, eds. *Brenner and Rector's The Kidney*. 10th ed. Philadelphia, PA: Elsevier; 2016.

Silverman SG, Pedrosa I, Ellis JH, et al. Bosniak classification of cystic renal masses, version 2019: an update proposal and needs assessment. *Radiology*. 2019;292(2):475-488. doi:10.1148/radiol.2019182646

Chapter 7
Clinical Pharmacology

王宗悅
祥佑診所

楊智宇
臺北榮民總醫院腎臟科

I. Diuretics

(I) Carbonic Anhydrase Inhibitor

PO: Acetazolamide 250 mg/tab	
Mechanism	Inhibit carbonic anhydrase in the proximal tubule
Indication	• Facilitate alkaline diuresis during alkalization therapy • Glaucoma • Acute mountain sickness prophylaxis: 250–750 mg QD • Prophylaxis of hypokalemic periodic paralysis • Idiopathic intracranial hypertension
Adverse effect	• Metabolic acidosis, hypokalemia, weakness, lethargy, abnormal taste, paresthesia, gastrointestinal distress, decreased libido • ↑ risk of nephrolithiasis
Reference	[1]

(II) Loop Diuretics

- PO: Furosemide 40 mg/tab, Bumetanide 1 mg/tab
- Intravenous (IV): Furosemide 20 mg, Bumetanide 0.5 mg/mL (4 mL/amp)

Mechanism	• Inhibit sodium-potassium-chloride cotransporter (NKCC2) in thick ascending limb Impairing urine concentration *Diuretic braking phenomenon: Post-diuretic renal salt retention and compensatory distal reabsorption *Ceiling effect: Increasing a diuretic dose above the ceiling does not increase the maximal minute-natriuresis
Indication	Edematous condition: ➢ Heart failure ➢ Liver cirrhosis ➢ Nephrotic syndrome Non-edematous condition: ➢ Hypercalcemia ➢ Hyperkalemia

Ceiling IV dose (mg)	Preserved renal function (estimated glomerular filtration rate [eGFR] > 75 min/mL)			Renal insufficiency	
	Nephrotic syndrome	Liver cirrhosis	Heart failure	Moderate GFR 20–50	Severe GFR < 20
	Furosemide				
	80–120	40–80	40–80	80–160	200
	Bumetanide				
	3	1	1	6	10

Adverse effect	Hypokalemia, hypochloremic alkalosis, hyperuricemia, hypocalcemia, hypomagnesemia, ototoxicity
Reference	[1,2]

(III) Thiazide

PO: hydrochlorothiazide 50 mg/tab, indapamide 1.5 mg/tab	
Mechanism	Inhibit thiazide-sensitive sodium chloride cotransporter (NCC) in distal convoluted tubule
Indication	Nephrolithiasis, diabetes insipidus, combination use with loop diuretics, osteoporosis
Dosing	
Adverse effect	Hyponatremia, hypercalcemia
Reference	[1]

(IV) Potassium-Sparing Diuretics, Mineral Corticoid Receptor Antagonist (MRA)

• Non-selective: spironolactone 25 mg/tab • Selective: eplerenone 50 mg/tab, finerenone	
Mechanism	Inhibit luminal Na^+ entry via amiloride-sensitive sodium channel on the cells in the late distal convoluted tubule, connecting tubule, and cortical collecting duct
Indication	• Hypokalemic alkalosis, especially in combination with a thiazide diuretic treat hypertension associated with hyperaldosteronism and for resistant hypertension • Spironolactone: cirrhotic ascites, heart failure with reduced ejection fraction • Eplerenone is indicated to prevent cardiac remodeling and systolic dysfunction setting of recent myocardial infarction • Finerenone therapy improved cardiovascular outcomes as compared with placebo in patients with type 2 diabetes and stage 2–4 chronic kidney disease (CKD) with moderately elevated albuminuria or stage 1 or 2 CKD with severely elevated albuminuria
Adverse effect	• Hyperkalemia • Gynecomastia may occur in men (lower risk in selective MRA)
Reference	[1,3]

(V) Sodium/Glucose Cotransporter 2 (SGLT2) Inhibitor

	Empagliflozin, dapagliflozin, canagliflozin		
Mechanism	Block glucose reabsorption in the proximal tubule, thereby delivering much of the filtered glucose to the urine and inducing an osmotic diuresis		
Indication	Used in patients with type 2 diabetes as glucose-lowering therapies, with additional benefits of weight loss and blood pressure reduction		
	Canagliflozin CREDENCE)	Empagliflozin (EMPA-REG)	Dapagliflozin (DAPA-CKD)
Population			
GFR	30–90	> 30	25–75
Heart failure (HF)	14.9%	• Placebo: 10.5% • Empagliflozin: 9.9%	• Placebo: 10.8% • Dapagliflozin: 10.9%
Diabetes mellitus	All	All	• Placebo: 67.4% • Dapagliflozin: 67.6%
Established cardiovascular disease (CVD)	• Placebo: 50.3% • Canagliflozin: 50.5%	All	• Placebo: 37.0% • Dapagliflozin: 37.8%
Outcome			
Renal	• End-stage kindney disease (ESKD) onset • Creatinine × 2 ↑	N/A	ESKD onset > 50% eGFR ↓
	Lower risk		Lower risk
CVD	• 3-point major adverse cardiovascular events (MACE) • HF hospitalization	• 3-point MACE • HF hospitalization	• Death from CVD • HF hospitalization
	Lower risk	Lower risk	Lower risk
Adverse effect	• Polyuria (osmotic diuresis) • Fungal genital infections • Diabetic ketoacidosis • A higher rate of leg amputations with canagliflozin in the CANVAS trials		
Reference	[4-6]		

(VI) AST-120 (KREMEZIN®)

Mechanism	Oral, spherical carbon particles that adsorb uremic toxins and their precursors within the gastrointestinal tract			
Indication	Results from randomized controlled trials remain inconclusive in prolonging the time to initiation of dialysis in patients with progressive CKD			
	Trial	Population	Endpoint	Results
	CAP-KD (Japan)	Progressive CKD (serum creatinine [SCr] < 5.0 mg/dL with negative 1/Cr slope)	• SCr ×2 ↑ • SCr > 6 • Dialysis	No difference compared with placebo
	• EPPIC-1 • EPPIC-2 (North America Latin America, Europe)	• Moderate to severe CKD • SCr 2.0–5.0 for men and 1.5–5.0 for women	• SCr ×2 ↑ • Dialysis	No difference compared with placebo [post-hoc analysis] might delay the time to primary endpoint in CKD patients from the USA population
	K-STAR (Korea)	CKD stage 3 or 4.	• SCr ×2 ↑ • Dialysis	No difference compared with placebo
Reference	[7]			

II. Uremic Bleeding Related Medication

(I) Desmopressin

IV 4 mcg/1 mL/amp	
Mechanism	• Increasing the release of large factor VIII: von Willebrand factor multimers from endothelial cells • Improved platelet aggregation on contact with collagen and increased concentrations of platelet glycoprotein (GP) Ib/IX
Dosing	0.3 mcg/kg in 50 mL of saline over 15–30 minutes
Adverse effect	• Reduced urine volume • Hyponatremia
Reference	[8]

Chapter 7 Clinical Pharmacology

(II) Estrogen

• PO: 0.625 mg/tab	
• IV: 25 mg/amp	
Mechanism	Decreasing production of L-arginine → inhibition of vascular nitric oxide production → thromboxane A2 and adenosine diphosphate ↑ → platelet aggregation ↑
Dosing	• 2.5–25.0 mg orally per day • 0.6 mg/kg intravenously daily for five days
Adverse effect	Venous thromboembolism
Reference	[9]

III. Phosphate Binders

(I) Calcium Containing

• Calcium acetate 667 mg/tab (elemental Ca: 169 mg)	
• Calcium carbonate 500 mg/tab (elemental Ca: 200 mg)	
Mechanism	Reduce intestinal absorption of dietary phosphate
Indication	• If phosphorus or intact parathyroid hormone (iPTH) levels cannot be controlled within the target range, despite dietary phosphorus restriction, phosphate binders should be prescribed • Target range (Kidney Disease Outcomes Quality Initiative, KDOQI): ➢ CKD stage 3–4: 2.7–4.6 mg/dL ➢ CKD stage 5: 3.5–5.5 mg/dL
Dosing	• With meal • Elemental calcium provided by phosphate binder should not exceed 1,500 mg/day
Adverse effect	Hypercalcemia, extra-skeletal calcification, GI upset
Non-calcium containing:	
➢ Sevelamer hydrochloride 800 mg/tab	
➢ Sevelamer carbonate 800 mg/tab, 800 mg/pk	
➢ Lanthanum carbonate 500/750/1,000 mg/tab	
➢ Ferric citrate (nephoxil) 500 mg/cap	
Indication	• Preferred in dialysis patients with severe vascular and/or other soft tissue calcifications • Ferric citrate may be more suitable for the treatment of chronic hyperphosphatemia in CKD patients requiring iron supplements

Adverse effect	GI upset				
Equivalent dose					
Calcium acetate	Calcium carbonate	Sevelamer	Lanthanum carbonate	Ferric citrate	
667 mg	750 mg	800 mg	1,000 mg	640 mg	
Reference	[10,11]				

IV. Drugs to Treat Secondary Hyperparathyroidism

(I) Active Vitamin D

• 1α-hydroxyvitamin D3: Onealfa 0.5 mcg/tab	
• 1,25-dihydroxyvitamin D3: Macalol 0.25 mcg/cap	
Mechanism	1,25-(OH)2 D3 has been shown to inhibit PTH gene transcription and to block parathyroid cell hyperplasia
Indication	CKD stage 5D with serum levels of intact PTH levels > 300 pg/mL should receive an active vitamin D sterol to reduce the serum levels of PTH to a target range of 150–300 pg/mL (KDOQI)
Adverse effect	Hypercalcemia, hyperphosphatemia
Reference	[12]

(II) Calcimimetics

Cinacalcet 25 mg/tab	
Etelcalcetide 2.5 mg/vial; 5 mg/vial	
Mechanism	Allosteric activators of the CaR, changing its structural conformation and stereo-selectively increasing sensitivity to extracellular Ca2+
Indication	As described in active form vitamin D
Adverse effect	Hypocalcemia, hypophosphatemia, GI upset
Reference	[10]

V. Drugs to Treat Renal Anemia

(I) Erythropoietin-Stimulating Agents

Erythropoietin-stimulating agents		Half-life (hr)	
Route		Subcutaneous	IV
Epotin α (Eprex) 2,000 IU		19.4	6.8
Epotin β (Recormon) 2,000 IU		24.2	8.8
Darbepoetin α (NESP) 20 mcg		48.8	25.3
Methoxy polyethylene glycol-epoetin beta (MIRCERA) 50 mcg; 100 mcg		133	130
Mechanism	• Erythropoiesis-stimulating agents (ESAs) stimulate erythropoiesis by activating erythropoietin receptors		
Indication	• For adult CKD 5D patients, ESA therapy is used to avoid having the hemoglobin (Hb) concentration fall below 9.0 g/dL by starting ESA therapy when the Hb is between 9.0–10.0 g/dL		
	• In general, ESAs are not used to maintain Hb concentration above 11.5 g/dL in adult patients with CKD (KDIGO)		
Adverse effect	• thromboembolic events are increased		
	• hypertension		
Iron	• IV: Ferric hydroxide 2,000 mg/5 mL/vial (Fe: 100 mg)		
	• PO: Ferrous citrate (Fe: 50 mg)		
Indication	For adult CKD patients with anemia not on iron or ESA therapy, we suggest a trial of IV iron (or in CKD ND patients, alternatively, a 1–3 month trial of oral iron therapy) if:		
	➢ An increase in Hb concentration without starting ESA treatment is desired AND.		
	➢ Transferrin saturation is $\leq$ 30% and ferritin is $\leq$ 500 ng/mL ($\leq$ 500 µg/L)		
Adverse effect	• Hypotensive and/or anaphylactoid reactions (mainly semilabile iron-sugar complexes such as iron sucrose and iron gluconate)		
	• Risk or infections		
Reference	[13]		

(II) Hypoxia-Inducible Factor (HIF) Stabilizer

Roxadustat (EVRENZO®)	
Mechanism	• HIF-α subunit dimerizes with HIF-β, moves to the cellular nucleus, and activates erythropoietin synthesis • Prolyl hydroxylase domains (PHDs) hydroxylate the HIF-α subunit leading to its polyubiquitination and subsequent proteasomal degradation • HIF stabilizer is an inhibitor of HIF-PHD
Indication	• Authorization for roxadustat in China for the treatment of anemia caused by CKD in non-dialysis-dependent (NDD) patients, as well as those who are dialysis-dependent (DD) in 2019 • Japan's Ministry of Health, Labor and Welfare (MHLW) approved roxadustat for the treatment of anemia associated with CKD in dialysis patients in 2019, and for the treatment of anemia of CKD in adult patients not on dialysis in 2020 • The US Food and Drug Administration (FDA) does not support approval for the treatment of anemia in CKD in DD adult patients in 2021
Reference	[1,14,15]

References

[1] Yu ASL, Chertow GM, Luyckx VA, Marsden PA, Skorecki K, Taal MW, eds. *Brenner and Rector's The Kidney.* 11th ed. Philadelphia, PA: Elsevier; 2019.

[2] Brater DC. Diuretic therapy. *N Engl J Med.* 1998;339(6):387-395. doi:10.1056/NEJM199808063390607

[3] Pitt B, Filippatos G, Agarwal R, et al. Cardiovascular events with finerenone in kidney disease and type 2 diabetes. *N Engl J Med.* 2021;385(24):2252-2263. doi:10.1056/NEJMoa2110956

[4] Perkovic V, Jardine MJ, Neal B, et al. Canagliflozin and renal outcomes in type 2 diabetes and nephropathy. *N Engl J Med.* 2019;380(24):2295-2306. doi:10.1056/NEJMoa1811744

[5] Zinman B, Wanner C, Lachin JM, et al. Empagliflozin, cardiovascular outcomes, and mortality in Type 2 diabetes. *N Engl J Med.* 2015;373(22):2117-2128. doi:10.1056/NEJMoa1504720

[6] Heerspink HJL, Stefánsson BV, Correa-Rotter R, et al. Dapagliflozin in patients with chronic kidney disease. *N Engl J Med.* 2020;383(15):1436-1446. doi:10.1056/NEJMoa2024816

[7] Asai M, Kumakura S, Kikuchi M. Review of the efficacy of AST-120 (KREMEZIN®) on renal function in chronic kidney disease patients. *Ren Fail.* 2019;41(1):47-56. doi:10.1080/0886022X.2018.1561376

[8] Hong SY, Yang DH. Effect of deamino-8-D-arginine desmopressin in uremic bleeding. *Korean J Intern Med.* 1996;11(2):145-150. doi:10.3904/kjim.1996.11.2.145

[9] Hedges SJ, Dehoney SB, Hooper JS, Amanzadeh J, Busti AJ. Evidence-based treatment

recommendations for uremic bleeding. *Nat Clin Pract Nephrol*. 2007;3:138-153. doi:10.1038/ncpneph0421

[10] National Kidney Foundation. K/DOQI clinical practice guidelines for bone metabolism and disease in chronic kidney disease. *Am J Kidney Dis*. 2003;42(4 Suppl 3):S1-S201.

[11] Daugirdas JT, Blake PG, Ing TS, eds. Handbook of Dialysis. 5th ed. Philadelphia, PA: Wolters Kluwer Health; 2015.

[12] Kidney Disease: Improving Global Outcomes (KDIGO) CKD-MBD Work Group. KDIGO clinical practice guideline for the diagnosis, evaluation, prevention, and treatment of Chronic Kidney Disease-Mineral and Bone Disorder (CKD-MBD). *Kidney Int Suppl*. 2009;(113):S1-S130. doi:10.1038/ki.2009.188

[13] Matzke GR. Intravenous iron supplementation in end-stage renal disease patients. *Am J Kidney Dis*. 1999;33(3):595-597. doi:10.1016/s0272-6386(99)70199-x

[14] Fishbane S, Spinowitz B. Update on anemia in ESRD and earlier stages of CKD: core curriculum 2018. *Am J Kidney Dis*. 2018;71(3):423-435. doi:10.1053/j.ajkd.2017.09.026

[15] Wyatt CM, Drüeke TB. HIF stabilization by prolyl hydroxylase inhibitors for the treatment of anemia in chronic kidney disease. *Kidney Int*. 2016;90(5):923-925. doi:10.1016/j.kint.2016.08.016

Chapter 8
Common Problems in Hemodialysis Patients

陳紀瑜
臺北榮民總醫院腎臟科
林堯彬
臺北榮民總醫院腎臟科

一、Timing for Hemodialysis (HD) Initiation

（一）Chronic kidney disease (CKD) 病患之 glomerular filtration rate (GFR) < 30 mL/min/1.73 m^2（即 stage 4 或以上）時，即應衛教告知 renal replacement therapy 之種類與優劣 [1]。

（二）CKD 病患開始長期血液透析 (maintenance HD) 之時機，應考量尿毒症症狀，而非 GFR 低於某特定閾值即需透析 [1]。

（三）Acute kidney injury 病患若出現 life-threatening hyperkalemia, metabolic acidosis, pulmonary edema 或其他 uremic complications 即需透析 [2]。

（四）尿毒症之症狀如 Table 8-1 所示，而 protein-energy wasting、fluid overload、seizure, encephalopathy、pericarditis, refractory hyperkalemia、metabolic acidosis 以及 uremic bleeding 為常見需透析之適應症 [3]。

（五）2010 Initiating Dialysis Early and Late (IDEAL) study [4] 發現，GFR 10–15 mL/min/1.73 m^2 (by Cockcroft-Gault equation [C-G equation]) 之 CKD 病患，若無尿毒症症狀，early-start group (mean GFR at HD initiation: 12.0 by C-G equation; 9.0 by modification of diet in renal disease [MDRD] equation) 與 late-start group (mean GFR at HD initiation: 9.8 by C-G equation; 7.8 by MDRD equation) 相比，兩組之 all-cause mortality、cardiovascular events、infection、dialysis complications 均無差異。

（六）過去十年來，臺灣 CKD 病患開始接受透析時的 median estimated glomerular filtration rate (eGFR) 為 5 mL/min/1.73 m^2 (range 3–11 mL/min/1.73 m^2 by MDRD equation)。

Table 8-1. 尿毒症之症狀 (symptoms) 與徵兆 (sign)

症狀	徵兆
虛弱、疲倦	癲癇發作
意識混亂 (confusion)	無月經
噁心想吐	中心體溫 (core temperature) 降低
嗅覺味覺改變	蛋白質熱量耗損 (protein-energy wasting)
睡眠障礙	胰島素阻抗 (insulin resistance)
皮膚搔癢	肋膜炎
痙攣 (cramps)	心包膜炎
不寧腿	打嗝
	血小板功能不良 (platelet dysfunction)

二、Vascular Access in HD

（一）Type of Vascular Access

1. Arteriovenous Fistula (AVF)

(1) 自體靜脈以手術連接至動脈，經 1–3 個月後，待「arterialized vein」形成後，可供 HD 上針透析用 [3,5]。

(2) 優點
- A. Lowest thrombosis rate.
- B. Longer survival.
- C. Lower infection rate.

(3) 缺點
- A. Long maturation time.
- B. Requirement of adequate vein.
- C. Possible failure to mature.
- D. Cosmetically unattractive.

(4) Brescia-Cimino radio-cephalic AVF：1966 年發明，side-to-side anastomosis。目前則改為 end of cephalic vein to side of radial artery，可避免 venous hypertension 及維持 distal flow in artery (Figure 8-1)。

(5) Wrist (radiocephalic) AVF 最佳，elbow (brachiocephalic) AVF 次之，upper arm (brachiobasilic) AVF 最末。Brachiobasilic vein 因 basilic vein 位於深處，需 transposition (superficialization) 至表淺皮膚下。

Type of AVF

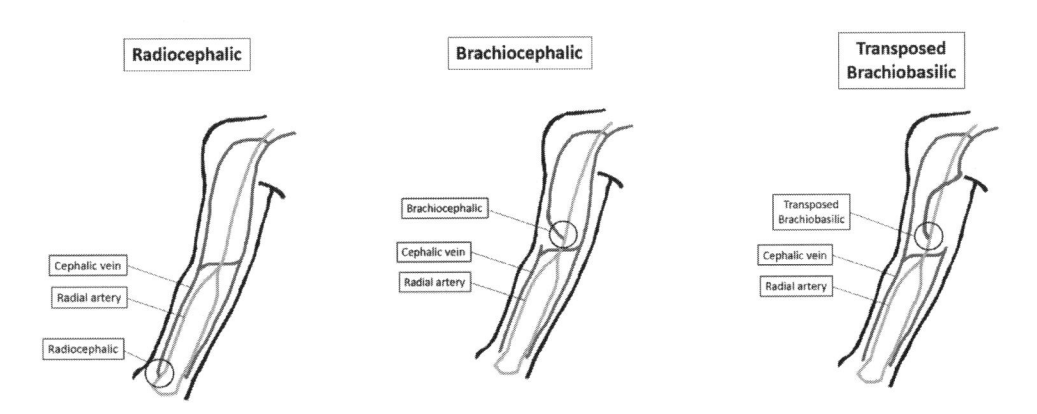

Figure 8-1. Types of arteriovenous fistula (AVF)

2. Arteriovenous graft (AVG)

(1) 植入一 expanded polytetrafluoroethylene 材質之人工血管，做為上針透析用 (Figure 8-2) [3,5]。

(2) 優點

　　A. Ease of placement.

　　B. Short time between placement and cannulation (2 weeks).

　　C. Not require an adequate vein.

　　D. Low early thrombosis rate.

(3) 缺點

　　A. Higher infection rate.

　　B. One-year primary patency rate (只有 50%) [3].

3. Tunneled-Cuffed Catheter

(1) Tunneled：導管進入皮膚後，會有一段距離處於皮下組織間 (tunneled) 才進入血管。Cuffed：導管上有一 Dacron cuff。這兩點均可降低感染率 [3,5]。

(2) 優點

　　A. Immediate use.

　　B. Unnecessity of skin puncture.

　　C. Little change of high-cardiac output heart failure.

(3) 缺點

　　A. Low blood flow rate.

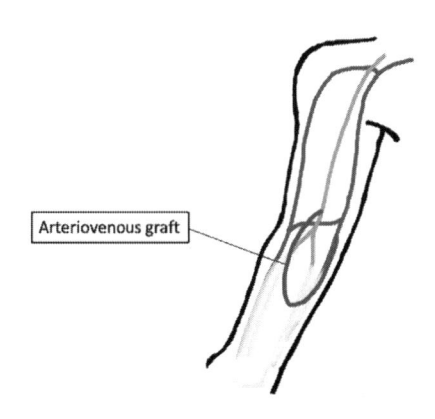

Figure 8-2. Arteriovenous (AV) graft

B. Higher infection rate compared to AVF or AVG.
C Higher thrombosis rate.
D. Risk of pulmonary or pericardial complications.
E. Risk of central venous stenosis.

4. Non-Tunneled Catheter
(1) 無 cuff，做為緊急透析用。
(2) 可置放於 internal jugular vein 或 femoral vein。不建議置放於 subclavian vein，易增加日後中央靜脈狹窄風險。

（二）Preparation of Vascular Access

1. 預期「一年內」會進入血液透析，即可考慮建立 AVF [1]。
2. 當 eGFR 15–20 mL/min/1.73 m2 (MDRD equation)，可考慮建立 AVF [5]。

（三）Complications of Vascular Access

Thrombosis and Stenosis:
1. AVF/AVG：當 thrill 與 bruit 減弱或消失，血管通路遠端肢體腫漲，上針時抽出血塊，透析後不易止血，血管通路血流不足都是血管通路阻塞的徵兆。
   (1) 預防方法：dipyridamole 加上 aspirin 可預防 AVG 阻塞。遠紅外線照射可預防 AVF 阻塞。Clopidogrel 及 fish oil 效果不佳。不建議預防性 angioplasty。
   (2) 治療方法：thrombectomy 加上 percutaneous transluminal angioplasty。
2. Dialysis catheter：血液無法抽出或流量下降即為阻塞。
   (1) 預防方法：僅小型研究發現 citrate-locking solution 有效。High-dose heparin locking solution，systemic warfarin 均無效。
   (2) 治療方法：更換導管。

三、足量透析 (HD Adequacy)

（一）Definition：消除病患尿毒症狀、達最佳存活率之最小透析量

1. Adequacy of dialysis 不代表 adequacy of patient care。照顧透析病患目標除達到足量透析外，也需處理貧血、營養、腎性骨病變、血糖、血脂、心血管疾病及心理問題 [1]。

2. 評估透析劑量 (dialysis dose) 以小分子清除率（如 urea）最為重要，包含 Kt/V 與 urea reduction ratio (URR)。
3. Kidney Disease: Improving Global Outcomes (KDIGO) 準則建議，若病患接受每週三次 HD，每次透析之 Kt/V 需 ≥ 1.2，目標為 1.4 [1]。
4. $URR = \dfrac{PreHD\ BUN - PostHD\ BUN}{PostHD\ BUN} \times 100\%$
5. URR 代表每次透析所能移除的尿素氮比率，需大於 65%–70%。因無法計算病患尿素分布體積 (V)、透析時尿素產生量與腎臟殘餘尿素清除率，故目前準則已不建議使用 [1]。
6. Kt/V，代表 fractional urea clearance，為目前評估 dialysis dose 最常用的指標。K：透析器之尿素清除率，單位為 mL/min or L/hr。t：透析時間, 單位為 min or hr。V：病患之尿素分布體積，單位為 mL or L。因此 Kt/V = 1.0 即表示該次透析治療所清除乾淨之血液體積等於病患之尿素分布體積。
7. Kt/V = –ln (R – 0.008 × T) + (4 – 3.5 × R) × ultrafiltration (UF)/W
   R: Post-HD blood urea nitrogen (BUN)/Pre-HD BUN.
   T：透析時間（單位：hr）。
   UF：透析脫水量（單位：kg）。
   W：透析後體重（單位：kg）。
8. Kidney Disease Outcomes Quality Initiative 的 2006 年足量透析指引建議：不論 Kt/V 值多高，若患者殘餘尿量很少或沒有，透析時間均不應低於 3 小時（對每週透析 3 次者而言）。

四、Acute Complications of HD Patients

透析中常見之併發症依發生的頻率依序為 hypotension (Table 8-2)、cramps、nausea/vomiting、headache、chest pain、back pain、itching [3,6]。

（一）Hypotension

1. 緊急處理方式
(1) 頭低腳高左側躺的姿勢 (trendelenburg position)。
(2) UF 速率應盡可能降至零。
(3) 注射 0.9% 生理食鹽水（100 mL 或更多）或 hypertonic solution（如：D50W、mannitol、albumin）。

Table 8-2. Causes of intradialytic hypotension

Causes of intradialytic hypotension
1. Volume related
a. Large interdialytic weight gain (high ultrafiltration rate)
b. Short dialysis (high ultrafiltration rate)
c. Low target ("dry") weight
d. Nonvolumetric dialysis (inaccurate or erratic ultrafiltration)
e. Low dialysis solution [Na+] (intracellular fluid shift)
2. Inadequate vasoconstriction
a. High dialysis solution temperature
b. Autonomic neuropathy
c. Antihypertensive medications
d. Eating during treatment
e. Anemia
f. Acetate buffer
3. Cardiac factors
a. Diastolic dysfunction
b. Arrhythmia (atrial fibrillation)
c. Ischemia
4. Uncommon causes
a. Pericardial tamponade
b. Myocardial infarction
c. Occult hemorrhage
d. Septicemia
e. Dialyzer reaction
f. Hemolysis
g. Air embolism

2. 預防方法

(1) 降低 interdialytic weight gain，勿大於體重之 5%。

(2) 設定適當乾體重 (dry weight)。

(3) 透析前停止服用降血壓藥物。

(4) 降低透析液溫度，35.5°C 或設定為比患者透析前的耳溫低 0.5°C。

(5) 若還有相當的殘餘腎功能，考慮使用利尿劑來增加尿量。

(6) 避免於透析過程進食。

(7) 透析前血紅素值維持 10–11 g/dL。

(8) 若 UF 速率 > 13 mL/kg/hr，要增加每週的透析總時數。

(9) 使用 midodrine。
(10) 對自主神經異常導致透析低血壓，可考慮用升壓劑 sertraline。
(11) 考慮嘗試使用血液容積監視器 (blood volume monitor)。
(12) Refractory intradialytic hypotension 的病患，在可忍受下，考慮使用鈉濃度較高的 (140–145 mmol/L) 的透析液。

（二）Muscle Cramps

1. 處理方式

(1) 治療可能伴隨之透析中低血壓。
(2) 提高透析液鈉濃度至恰好低於引發透析後乾渴感的界線值。
(3) 避免透析前鉀、鈣、鎂濃度過低。
(4) 注射 hypertonic solution（如 3% saline、D50W、mannitol）。
(5) 用力伸展患側肌肉。
(6) 血行動力學穩定病患可考慮使用 nifedipine 10 mg。
(7) 補充肉鹼 (carnitine) 可能可減少透析間的抽筋。
(8) 雖然透析前服用 Quinine sulfate 來避免透析中抽筋相當有效，但因為副作用多（thrombocytopenia、QTc prolong、過敏反應），現在已不建議用來預防抽筋 [6]。

（三）Nausea and Vomiting

1. 原因

(1) 大部分與低血壓有關。
(2) 也有可能是不平衡症候群的早期表現。
(3) A/B 型的透析膜效應 (dialyzer reaction)。
(4) 糖尿病患胃輕癱 (gastroparesis) 因透析加重。

2. 處置

(1) 處理與任何低血壓相關事件，小心 aspiration 的發生。
(2) 避免透析中發生低血壓。
(3) 若症狀持續且與血流動力學無關，透析前單次給予 Metoclopramide (primperan) 5–10 mg 可能有效。

（四）Headache

1. 原因

(1) 病因大部分未明。
(2) 可能是不平衡症候群的輕微表現。
(3) 透析可能使偏頭痛患者復發。
(4) 非典型或特別劇烈的頭痛，應排除神經學上的原因。

2. 處置

透析中給 acetaminophen。

（五）Chest Pain and Back Pain

1. 原因

(1) 1%–4% 透析治療會發生輕微的胸痛或不適（常與背痛相連），原因未明。
(2) 或許更換另一種透析器會有幫助。
(3) 需與其他可能引發胸痛原因做鑑別診斷。

（六）Itching

1. 原因

(1) 確保足量透析，Kt/V ≥ 1.2。
(2) 鈣磷乘積升高或 parathyroid hormone (PTH) 大幅升高者。
(3) 若癢只出現在透析期間，特別是有合併其他輕微過敏症狀，可能是對透析器或血液迴路管低度過敏表現。

2. 處置

(1) 長期使用潤膚劑 (emollients) 全面保濕和潤滑皮膚。
(2) 第一線：抗組織胺。
(3) 第二線：Gabapentin 或 pregabalin、UBV、口服活性碳或 Nalfurafine。
(4) 若還是無效：Naltrexone、tacrolimus 藥膏。

（七）Dialysis Disequilibrium Syndrome

1. 症狀

(1) 輕微：nausea and vomiting、headaches、fatigue、restlessness。
(2) 嚴重：mental change、generalized seizure、coma。

(3) 因為 earlier initiation of maintenance HD，所以目前已大幅減少 dialysis disequilibrium syndrome。

2. 原因

(1) Reverse urea theory:
    BUN 雖是 ineffective osmole，但也需數小時才能平衡。尿毒症病患腦中的 urea transporter 下降，aquaporin 上升，故透析時腦細胞內的 BUN 濃度較血液中來得高，促使水分進入腦細胞，造成 brain swelling。
(2) Paradoxical acidosis in cerebrospinal fluid: diffusion of carbon dioxide across blood-brain barrier [3].

3. 預防

(1) Timely initiation of dialysis.（最重要）
(2) Use of a small surface-area dialyzer.（不要洗得太乾淨）
(3) Low blood flow.
(4) Reducing dialysate flow or using current (versus counter-current).
(5) Increasing dialysate [Na+] or dialysate glucose or administering mannitol.

4. 治療：

(1) 停止透析。
(2) 輸注 mannitol。

五、Chronic Complications of HD Patients

（一）Cardiovascular Disease (CVD)

1. Cardiovascular disease (CVD) 是 HD 病患致死原因第一名，然而矯正 traditional risk factor（如 hyperlipidemia、inflammation、diabetes、hypertension、smoking、sedentary lifestyle、obesity），卻無法改善預後 [3]。
2. HD 病患有其他 nontraditional cardiovascular risk factors，如 chronic inflammation、genetic predisposition、oxidative stress、endothelial dysfunction、carbonyl stress 以及 accumulation of advanced glycation end-products。
3. 大規模研究證實不管是在一般大眾或透析病患，使用 folic acid 下降 homocysteine，

並無法改善 cardiovascular risk。但因為可以預防 nutritional deficiency 和 facilitate hematopoiesis，故還是會使用 folic acid。

4. Diagnosis of CVD in HD patients

    (1) Asymptomatic patients on HD 即可能有輕微 Troponin 上升。

    (2) Cardiac troponin T：most accurate prognostic indicator of cardiovascular events in HD，但是對於 acute coronary syndrome 預測效果不好。

5. 治療：

    (1) 「Die Deutsche Diabetes Dialyse Studie (4D study): Type 2 diabetes mellitus, HD」：雖然 atorvastatin 可以降低 42% low-density lipoprotein (LDL)，但是並沒有減少 primary endpoints of cardiovascular death、nonfatal myocardial infarction 以及 stroke；甚至 fatal stroke 還有上升的情形。

    (2) 「A study to evaluate the use of rosuvastatin in subjects on regular haemodialysis: an assessment of survival and cardiovascular events (AURORA study), HD」：rosuvastatin 無法改善血液透析病人之 cardiovascular deaths and nonfatal cardiovascular events，可能與 underlying cardiomyopathy 有關。

    (3) 「Acute coronary syndrome」依 United States Renal Data System 的 retrospective 分析，可能 coronary artery bypass graft 優於 percutaneous coronary intervention (PCI)。若做 PCI 的話，drug-eluting stent 較 bare metal stents 好，但未有 randomized controlled trial (RCT) 證實。

（二）Anemia

1. HD 病患因 erythropoietin 生成減少、紅血球壽命變短、透析時失血、尿毒素抑制紅血球生成、功能性鐵質缺乏、慢性炎症反應、鋁沉積、副甲狀腺高能症及藥物影響等因素，容易出現腎性貧血 [7]。

2. HD 病患宜至少「每月」檢測一次 hemoglobin (Hb)。

3. 有腎性貧血之 HD 病患宜檢測 complete blood count、absolute reticulocyte count、ferritin、transferrin saturation、serum vitamin B12、serum folate。

4. 成年 HD 病患，建議保持其血紅素值 > 9 g/dL；當血紅素值介於 9–10 g/dL 時，即可考慮使用血紅素生成刺激劑 (erythropoiesis stimulating agent, ESA)。

5. 成年 HD 病患均不應以 ESA 來維持血紅素值在 13 g/dL 以上。

6. 成年 HD 病患均不需例行性借助 ESA 來維持血紅素值在 11 g/dL 以上。

7. ESA 起始劑量應使血紅素值達每月上升 1–2 g/dL 速度，但不超過每月 2 g/dL。

8. ESA 起始劑量：

Epoetin-α 及 epoetin-β：20–50 U/kg BW/each time, TIW, SC or IV.

Darbepoetin-α：0.45 μg/kg BW, QW, SC or IV 或 0.75 μg/kg BW, Q2W, SC. Methoxy polyethylene glycol epoetin-β (Mircera)：0.6 μg/kg BW, Q2W, SC or IV.

9. ESA 反應不良：注射依體重計算之適當起始劑量的 ESA 一個月後，無法達到血紅素目標值或血紅素值上升幅度未超過 2%。最常見造成 ESA 反應不良的原因為鐵質缺乏，其他原因則包括維生素 B_{12} 缺乏、葉酸缺乏、甲狀腺低下症、使用 angiotensin-converting enzyme inhibitor/angiotensin II receptor blocker、感染、慢性炎症反應、溶血、活動性出血、腫瘤、營養不良、副甲狀腺亢進、單純紅血球再生不良 (pure red cell aplasia, PRCA)、血紅蛋白病 (hemoglobinopathy)、骨髓性疾病等。

10. PRCA：若 CKD 病人接受 ESA 超過八週，同時出現下列三種情形時，宜檢測抗體導致之 PRCA。

    (1) Hb 值以每週 0.5–1.0 g/dL 的速度下降或每一到二週即需輸血一次。

    (2) 網狀紅血球數目 (absolute reticulocyte count) 低於 10,000/μL。

    (3) 正常白血球及血小板數目。

    患有抗體導致之 PRCA 病人，應停用 ESA，並不應再使用任何紅血球生成素衍生之 ESA (Erythropoietin-derived ESA)，以免再誘發更多抗體。

11. 當 ferritin ≤ 500 ng/mL 或 transferrin saturation ≤ 30%，即可考慮使用鐵劑治療。

12. 在接受 ESA 合併鐵劑治療時，至少每三個月進行一次包括 ferritin 及 transferrin saturation 的鐵狀態評估。

13. HD 病患建議以靜脈注射為鐵劑使用途徑。

14. 若 HD 病人適合器官移植，建議儘量避免紅血球輸血，以減少 allo-immunization 風險。

15. 在發生以下臨床急性情況下，HD 病人接受紅血球輸血的好處可能大於風險：

    (1) 當病人有急性出血、不穩定性冠狀動脈疾病等情況時，必須快速矯正貧血以穩定病人病情。

    (2) 當緊急手術或介入性治療時，需即迅速矯正貧血。

16. 治療 HD 病人的慢性貧血，以下狀況可能紅血球輸血的好處大於風險：當紅血球生成刺激劑治療無效，例如地中海型貧血、鐮刀型血球性貧血、骨髓造血功能衰竭、紅血球生成刺激劑抗性等。

17. 紅血球生成刺激劑治療的風險可能超過其好處的情況有下列數種，例如以前或目前患有惡性腫瘤、中風病史等。

（三）Mineral Bone Disease in HD Patients

1. 腎性骨病變 (renal osteodystrophy) 為 CKD 病人骨骼系統形態上的改變，需利用骨切片的組織形態量測 [8]。

2. 當符合下列三種異常情況之一，皆可定義為 CKD 之礦物質骨異常 (mineral bone disease, MBD)：
   (1) 任何鈣離子、磷離子、副甲狀腺荷爾蒙及維他命 D 之代謝異常。
   (2) 任何骨骼之周轉、礦物質化、骨體積直線生長或骨強度異常。
   (3) 血管或其他軟組織之鈣化。
3. 透析病人應努力將升高之血清磷值下降至正常範圍：
   (1) 臨床檢驗室的正常血清磷值為 2.7–4.6 mg/dL。
   (2) 高血磷與 HD 病患之死亡率有正相關，開始血液透析病人使用磷結合劑，一年死亡率能降低約 25%。
   (3) 目前未有大型 RCT 確定透析病人血磷的最佳範圍。觀察型研究發現血磷 > 5.5 mg/dL 即可能與死亡率增加有關。
   (4) 現有口服磷結合劑（需餐中服用）：
       A. Calcium carbonate (500 mg)：1 g 的碳酸鈣與磷的結合能力大約與 1 g 醋酸鈣相同，而碳酸鈣內含 40% 的鈣。每日建議最高劑量的元素鈣為 1.5 g，因此碳酸鈣每日最多為 7.5 顆，副作用會高血鈣、噁心、便秘。
       B. Calcium acetate (667 mg)：1 g 降磷效果與 $CaCO_3$ 相當，但鈣只占了 25%，因此一天最多可以吃到 9 顆，副作用有高血鈣、噁心、便秘等。
       C. Sevelamer：800 mg 的 sevelamer 降磷效果與一顆 667 mg 醋酸鈣相當，價格較昂貴，可降低 LDL-C，副作用為噁心、腹瀉、消化不良。
       D. Lanthanum carbonate：降磷效果比鈣片好，價格昂貴，建議起始劑量為每日三次，每次 500 mg，依需要往上調整，但不建議每次超過 1,250 mg，副作用大多為腸胃道不適以及對長期安全性的質疑，但在後續的 1、3、6 年的報告均有良好的安全性。
       E. Ferric citrate：1 顆 500 mg 的檸檬酸鐵內含 105 mg 的三價鐵，起始劑量建議 4 g 分三次，可上調至每日最大劑量每日 6 g。降磷外也可補鐵及降低紅血球生成刺激劑的需求。
       F. Calcium citrate：因增加腸胃道鋁吸收，故不建議使用。
       G. Aluminum hydroxide：降磷效果佳，但可能有鋁中毒、dementia、adynamic bone disease 風險。
4. 透析病人血鈣值應保持於正常範圍內：
   (1) 臨床檢驗室正常血清鈣值為 8.5–10.0 mg/dL 或 8.5–10.5 mg/dL。
   (2) 目前未有大型 RCT 確定透析病人血鈣的最佳範圍。觀察型研究發現血鈣 > 9.5 mg/dL 與 < 8.4 mg/dL 即可能與死亡率增加有關。
   (3) 使用含鈣的磷結合劑，元素鈣一天不宜超過 1,500 mg（約等同 7.5# calcium

carbonate 或 9# calcium acetate），再加上飲食或透析液所攝入的元素鈣，一天元素鈣總量不宜超過 2,000 mg。

(4) 透析液中的鈣離子含量應介於 2.5–3.0 mEq/L 間。

(5) 若 HD 病患出現高血鈣、血管鈣化、adynamic bone disease、low serum PTH，則應減少含鈣之磷結合劑與活性維他命 D3 之使用。

5. 透析病人血清副甲狀腺素值應維持在正常上限的 2–9 倍。

(1) 腎臟病患者因磷排出下降造成高血磷，進一步導致低血鈣及次發性副甲狀腺亢進症。血清 intact PTH (iPTH) 過高與透析病人死亡率呈正相關。

(2) 因血清副甲狀腺值易受檢測方式而影響，因此 2009 年 KDIGO 準則建議保持血清副甲狀腺值於正常上限之 2–9 倍間。

(3) 次發性副甲狀腺高能亢進症之治療：

　A. 控制血磷：高血磷為 CKD-MBD 的根本原因。

　B. 活性維他命 D3：包含 calcitriol、alfacalcidol、paricalcitol，通常於每次透析後給予，較能符合生理性 calcitriol 濃度。常見劑量為 calcitriol 0.5–1.5 μg/HD session, paricalcitol 2–6 μg/HD session。副作用為造成高血鈣、高血磷與 adynamic bone disease。

　C. 擬鈣劑 (calcimimetic)：如 cinacalcet。目前常用劑量為 25–100 mg/day。價格昂貴。副作用為 nausea、vomiting、hypocalcemia。

參考文獻

[1] National Kidney Foundation. KDOQI clinical practice guideline for hemodialysis adequacy: 2015 update [published correction appears in Am J Kidney Dis. 2016;67(3):534]. *Am J Kidney Dis*. 2015;66(5):884-930. doi:10.1053/j.ajkd.2015.07.015

[2] Khwaja A. KDIGO clinical practice guidelines for acute kidney injury. *Nephron Clin Pract*. 2012;120(4):c179-c184. doi:10.1159/000339789

[3] Yu ASL, Chertow G, Luyckx VA, Marsden PA, Skorecki K, Taal MW, eds. *Brenner & Rector's the Kidney*. 11th ed. Philadelphia, PA: Elsevier; 2019.

[4] Cooper BA, Branley P, Bulfone L, et al. A randomized, controlled trial of early versus late initiation of dialysis. *N Engl J Med*. 2010;363(7):609-619. doi:10.1056/NEJMoa1000552

[5] Vascular Access 2006 Work Group. Clinical practice guidelines for vascular access. *Am J Kidney Dis*. 2006;48(Suppl 1): S176-S247. doi:10.1053/j.ajkd.2006.04.029

[6] Daugirdas JT, Blake PG, Ing TS, eds. *Handbook of Dialysis*. 5th ed. Philadelphia, PA: Wolters Kluwer Health; 2015.

[7] Summary of recommendation statements. *Kidney Int Suppl (2011)*. 2012;2(4):283-287.

doi:10.1038/kisup.2012.41

[8] Kidney Disease: Improving Global Outcomes (KDIGO) CKD-MBD Work Group. KDIGO clinical practice guideline for the diagnosis, evaluation, prevention, and treatment of chronic kidney disease-mineral and bone disorder (CKD-MBD). *Kidney Int Suppl.* 2009;(113):S1-S130. doi:10.1038/ki.2009.188

Chapter 9
Common Problems in Peritoneal Dialysis Patients

陳範宇
臺北榮民總醫院腎臟科
陳進陽
臺北榮民總醫院腎臟科

一、基礎概念 (Basic Concepts)

（一）Peritoneal membrane is semipermeable（半透膜）
（二）In peritoneal dialysis (PD):
1. the peritoneal membrane = dialysis membrane.
2. the peritoneal cavity = dialysate compartment.

（三）PD 的原理？
1. PD 是一種腎臟替代療法 (renal replacement therapy)。
2. 以病人的腹膜和微血管作為 blood 和 infused dialysis solution 之間的半透膜行水分和毒素的清除。

（四）PD 和 hemodialysis (HD) 何者對腎友的存活率有幫助？
　　PD 和 HD 兩者對於存活率上沒有顯著差異。

二、PD 的禁忌症 (PD Contraindications)

　　PD 的相對和絕對禁忌症：
（一）出現 uncorrectable mechanical defects（無法修復的腹部疝氣）。
（二）近期有接受 intra-abdominal surgery（包含 aortic vascular graft）。
（三）頻繁的 diverticulitis 或 intra-abdominal infections。
（四）Abdominal wall cellulitis.
（五）過去重複接受腹部手術並有 adhesion formation。
（六）病人無法自己正確操作換液步驟，且家中無其他適合的照顧者。

三、PD 導管 (PD Catheter)

（一）PD catheter segments = Intraperitoneal (IP) + Two-cuff tunnel + Extraperitoneal.
（二）Two-cuff = Deep cuff and subcutaneous cuff (Figure 9-1).
（三）最常被使用的 PD 導管？
　　Tenckhoff Catheter: two-cuff, silastic, intraperitoneal catheter.
（四）不同的 PD 導管在臨床功效上是否有差異？
　　No shape has proven more efficacious than another.
（五）臨床上有哪幾種導管植入法？

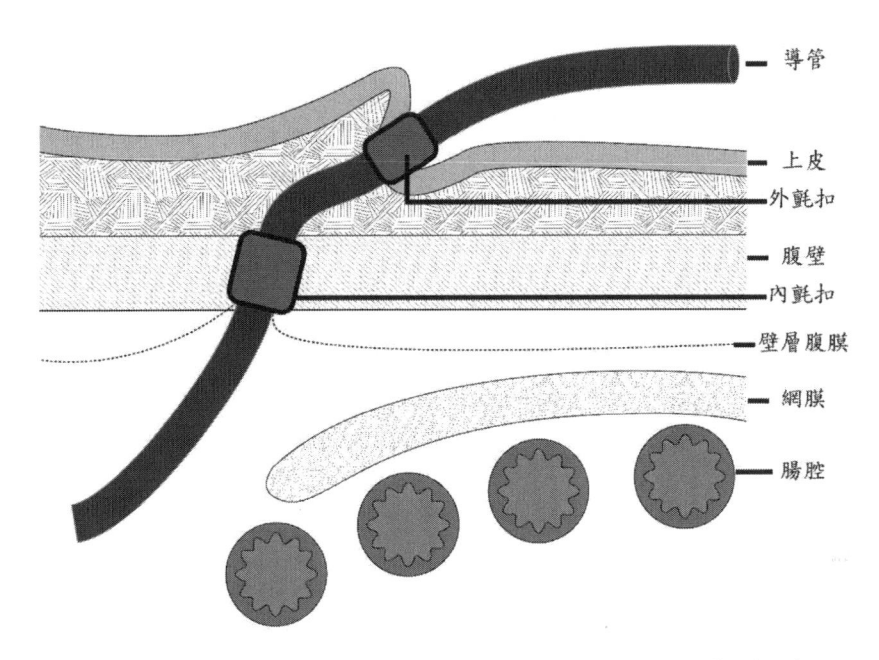

Figure 9-1. Peritoneal dialysis catheter and infectious complications[a]

[a] 資料參考來源：[1]。

Laparoscopic placement 或 percutaneous insertion. Open surgical placement of PD catheters 已經不再被常規執行。

（六）Percutaneous PD catheter insertion 有何優點？

植管時間短（約 30–60 分鐘），且可在植管後早期進行灌液，不需等待兩週。

（七）The Y-set and Flush-before-Fill Technique:
1. The Y-set is the standard setup in manual PD.
2. The flush-before-fill technique（先沖再灌）is where the patient flushes air first out of the tubing by allowing a small amount of dialysis solution to pass into the drain bag; the drain bag is then clamped and the rest of the dialysis solution is infused into the peritoneal cavity via gravity（過程約 10–15 分鐘）(Figure 9-2).

四、腹膜透析液 (PD Solutions)

（一）PD 液的三大組成？
1. An osmotic agent to induce ultrafiltration (UF).
2. A buffer to correct uremic metabolic acidosis.
3. A combination of electrolytes to optimize diffusive removal of solutes.

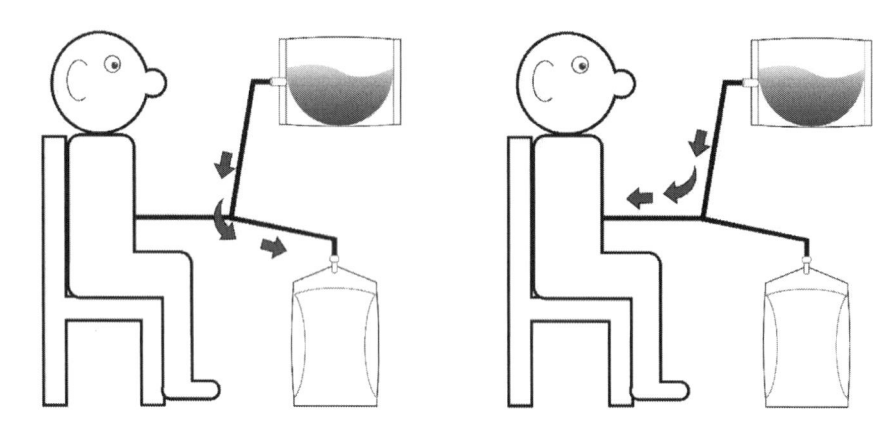

Figure 9-2. The Y-set and flush-before-fill technique[a]

[a] 資料參考來源：[2]。

（二）Standard PD solutions (dianeal) 包含 sodium、chloride、lactate、magnesium、calcium 和不同濃度的 dextrose (Table 9-1, Table 9-2)。

（三）7.5% Icodextrin (Extraneal) 健保給付規定（自 2019 年 8 月 1 日生效，每天限用一袋）

Table 9-1. Standard peritoneal dialysis solution components

Component	Concentration
Sodium, mEq/L	132
Potassium, mEq/L	None
Chloride, mEq/L	95–105
Calcium, mEq/L	2.5, 3.5
Phosphorus, mEq/L	None
Magnesium, mEq/L	1.5
Lactate, mEq/L	35, 40
Dextrose, %	1.50, 2.50, 4.25

Table 9-2. Standard peritoneal dialysis solution osmolarity[a]

Dextrose (%)	Glucose (g/dL)	Osmolarity (mOsm/L)
1.50	1.36	346
2.50	2.27	396
4.25	3.86	485

[a]Dextrose (glucose monohydrate) (molecular weight [MW]: 198) = Glucose (MW: 180) + H_2O (MW: 18).

1. High transporters 病患，用於每天長留置期。
2. High average transporters 病患，每天使用 1 袋 ≥ 2.5% 葡萄糖 PD 液。
3. 脫水衰竭病患及臨界脫水衰竭邊緣之病患，即病患下列情形之一者：
   (1) 使用 4.25% 傳統式葡萄糖 PD 液 4 小時內脫水量 ≤ 400 mL 者。
   (2) 每天使用總袋數 1/2 以上（含）≥ 2.5% 葡萄糖 PD 液。
   (3) glycated hemoglobin (HbA1c) > 7.0% 的糖尿病 PD 病患，用於每天長留置期。
   (4) 腹膜炎病患。

（四）為何 7.5% Icodextrin (Extraneal) 可能會導致病人不正確血糖判讀值？

因為 7.5% Icodextrin 會升高血糖中的麥芽糖濃度，所以只能使用具有葡萄糖專一性的血糖機或試紙 [3]。

（五）Nutrineal (1.1% amino acid) 健保給付規定（自 2010 年 5 月 1 日生效）
1. 限長期接受 PD 之病患使用；該病患至少接受 PD 三個月以上者。
2. 每天限使用一袋代替葡萄糖 PD 液。
3. Serum albumin ≤ 3.5 gm/dL 或 normalized protein nitrogen appearance < 0.9 患者使用，需附開始 CAPD 當月的檢驗報告影本。
4. 每週 Kt/V 需 > 1.7。
5. 不得同時合併其他胺基酸使用。

五、三孔模型 (The Three-Pore Model)

三孔模型 (Table 9-3) 包含 large pores、small pores 和 ultra-small pores。

Table 9-3. The three-pore model of peritoneal transport[a]

Pores	Size (nm)	Comments
Large	> 25	< 10% of solute removal (proteins and other macromolecules pass).
Small	4–6	> 90% of solute removal (electrolytes and solutes like urea and creatinine pass).
		60% of water transport
Ultra-small (Aquaporins)	0.3–0.5	AQP-1 (transport water only).
		40% of water transport (allowing only solute-free water to pass).

Abbreviation: AQP-1, aquaporin-1.

[a] 數量：Small > Ultra-small > Large pores.

六、腹膜平衡測驗 (Peritoneal Equilibration Test, PET)

（一）為何要做 PET ？

PET 可幫助病人決定其腹膜種類，協助醫護開立適合的 PD 處方。

（二）如何做 PET ？

1. An overnight dwell 8–12 hours is required and drain pretest exchange completely.
2. A 2-L infusion (200 mL/min for 10 min) of 2.5% dextrose solution is allowed to dwell for 4 hours.
3. Dialysis samples are taken after 0, 2, and 4 hours and analyzed for creatinine and glucose.
4. A serum sample is taken after 2 hours and analyzed for creatinine and glucose.
5. The dialysate-to-plasma (D/P) ratio of creatinine is calculated (D/P Cr).
6. The ratio of dialysate glucose at 4 hours to 0 hours is also calculated (D/D$_0$ Glu).

（三）Four classes of membrane transport characteristics are defined based on the rate of creatinine diffusion and glucose absorption (Figure 9-3, Table 9-4).

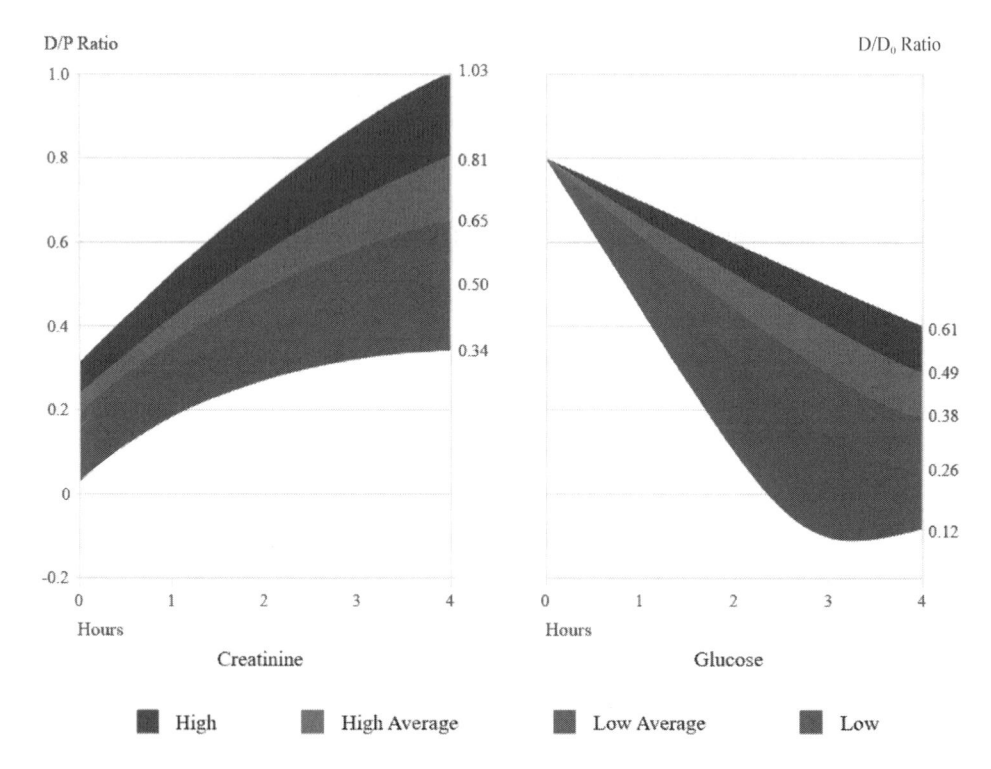

Figure 9-3. Peritoneal equilibration test-determined transport groups for dialysate-to-plasma ratio (D/P) of creatinine and dialysate-to-0 hour dialysate (D/D$_0$) of glucose[a]

[a] 資料參考來源：[4]。

Table 9-4. Peritoneal membrane types and characteristics

Membrane type	D/P Cr ratio	Characteristic
high	> 0.81	transport solutes quickly poor ultrafiltration protein loss
high average	0.65–0.81	transport solutes well adequate ultrafiltration
low average	0.5–0.64	transport solutes slowly good ultrafiltration
low	< 0.5	transport solutes slowly excellent ultrafiltration

Abbreviations: Cr, creatinine; D/P, dialysate-to-plasma ratio.

（四）高腹膜通透性和低腹膜通透性對腎友預後的差異？

The Canada-USA (CANUSA) Study Group 發現 high transport membranes 的病人有較高的 risk of technique failure 或 death。背後的可能機轉為：

1. Poor UF.（後續伴隨 hypertension 和 left ventricular hypertrophy）
2. Increased protein losses.

（五）何時要做 PET？

1. 首透後 4–8 週。
2. PET should be repeated when clinically indicated:
    (1) 出現無法解釋的體液容積過量。
    (2) 引流量減少。
    (3) 臨床上須使用更多的 hypertonic dialysate dwells 以維持引流量。
    (4) 高血壓惡化。
    (5) Change in measured peritoneal solute removal (Kt/Vurea).
    (6) Unexplained signs or symptoms of uremia.
3. PET 應在病人臨床穩定下再測量（距離腹膜炎完治後至少一個月以上）。

七、PD 的模式和處方開立 (PD Modalities and Prescription)

（一）PD 常見的模式詳見 Table 9-5 與 Figure 9-4。
（二）如何替腎友選擇 PD 的模式 (PD modality)？

先以 PET 決定其 peritoneal transport type，再選擇適合的處方 (Table 9-6)。

Table 9-5. Peritoneal dialysis 常見的模式

Modalities	Comments
連續性可攜帶腹膜透析 (CAPD)	Multiple exchanges during the day followed by a night dwell.
全自動腹膜透析 (APD)	A cycler performs multiple dwell.
連續循環式腹膜透析 (CCPD)	A cycler performs multiple night dwells followed by a day dwell.
每晚間歇式腹膜透析 (NIPD)	A cycler performs multiple night dwells; no day dwell is used.

Abbreviations: APD, automated peritoneal dialysis; CAPD, continuous ambulatory peritoneal dialysis; CCPD, continuous cyclic peritoneal dialysis; NIPD, nocturnal intermittent peritoneal dialysis.

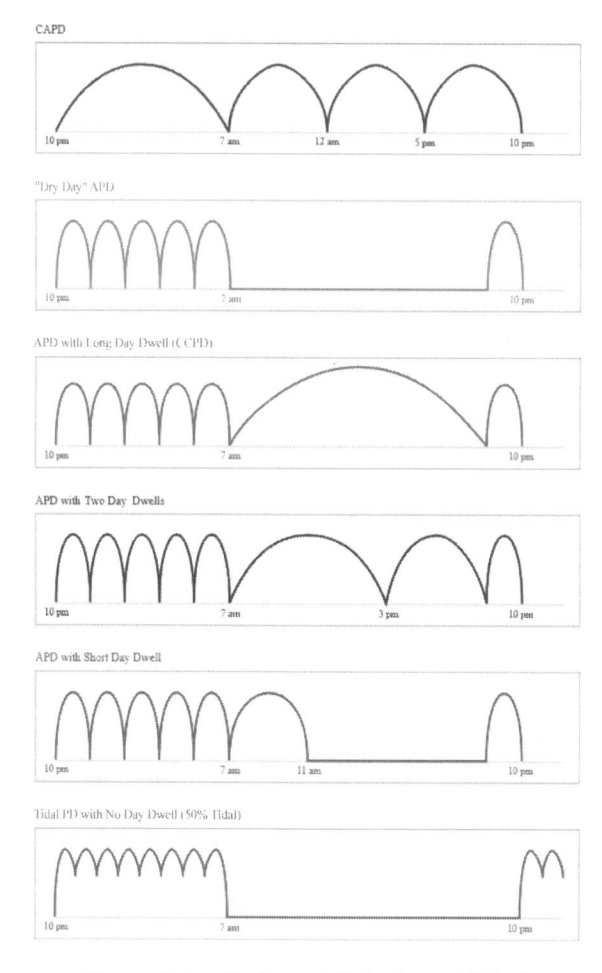

Figure 9-4. Peritoneal dialysis modalities[a]

Abbreviations: APD, automated peritoneal dialysis; CAPD, continuous ambulatory peritoneal dialysis; CCPD, continuous cyclic peritoneal dialysis.

[a] 資料參考來源：[2]。

Table 9-6. PD prescription recommendation

Transport type[a]	UF	Clearance	Prescription recommendation
High	Poor	Adequate	CCPD + Extraneal
High–average	Adequate	Adequate	CCPD
			Standard PD[b] + Extraneal
Low–average	Good	Inadequate-adequate	Standard PD[b]
			High-dose PD[c]
Low	Excellent	Inadequate	High-dose PD[c]
			HD

Abbreviations: CCPD, continuous cyclic peritoneal dialysis; HD, hemodialysis; PD, peritoneal dialysis; UF, ultrafiltration.

[a]High transporter：時間放短一點；Low transporter：時間放久一點＋量多一點。
[b]Standard PD: CAPD with 7.5–9.0 L/d, or CCPD with dialysis solution inflow 6–8 L overnight and 2 L daytime.
[c]High-dose PD: CAPD with > 9.0 L/d, or CCPD with inflow > 8 L overnight and/or 2 L daytime.

八、足量透析 (Dialysis Adequacy)

（一）Clearance Targets 為何？多久需測量一次是否達標？

1. The 2006 Kidney Disease Outcomes Quality Initiative (KDOQI) guidelines: A weekly clearance of urea (Kt/V_{urea}) of at least 1.7.
2. Clearance adequacy 應在開始接受 PD 後一個月檢測，並每四個月進行追蹤，或當病人臨床症狀有變化或是透析處方有更動時進行檢測。

（二）如何計算 Weekly Kt/V 與 Weekly Creatinine Clearance Rate (WCC)？

1. Weekly Kt/V_{urea} calculation = dialysis Kt/V_{urea} + renal Kt/V_{urea}
   Dialysis Kt/V_{urea} = (B)/(A)
   Renal Kt/V_{urea} = (C)/(A)
   (A) = volume of urea distribution (male: ideal body weight (IBW) × 0.6; female: ideal BW × 0.5)
   (B) = 24-hr D/P urea × 24-hr drained volume × 7
   (C) = 24-hr U/P urea × 24-hr urine volume × 7
2. Weekly CCR calculation = dialysis CCr L/week + renal CCr L/week
   Dialysis CCr L/week = 24-hr D/P Cr × 24-hr drained volume × 7 × (1.73 m^2/ body surface area [BSA])

Renal CCr L/week = [(24-hr U/P Cr) + (24-hr U/P urea)]/2 × 24-hr urine volume × 7 × (1.73 m^2/BSA)

（三）UF Targets 為何？

UF targets 較無明確定義，但 minimum of 750 mL of net fluid removal per day 在 anuric patients 有較佳的預後。

（四）何謂 Ultrafiltration Insufficiency (UFI)？

UFI is a condition of fluid overload in association with net UF of < 400 mL after a 4-hour dwell of 2 L of 4.25% dextrose.

（五）造成 UFI 的主要原因為何？

UFI 主因源於 peritoneal membrane dysfunction。臨床上主要有三大類腹膜功能異常 (Table 9-7 與 Figure 9-5) [5]。

1. 腹膜特性為 rapid small solute diffusion (fast peritoneal solute transfer rate)。
2. 腹膜特性為 poor intrinsic UF from the start of PD。
3. 腹膜特性 become less effective over time leading to acquired membrane insufficiency。

Table 9-7. Membrane dysfunction–classification, pathophysiology, recommendation

分類	病生理機轉	處置建議
Fast PSTR	1. 腹膜發炎。 2. 血管新生。	1. 若尚有餘尿功能：考慮 CAPD (dry nights) 或 APD (dry days)。 2. 考慮使用 icodextrin (daytime for APD, overnight for CAPD)。 3. 縮短 glucose-based 透析液的滯留時間。
Poor intrinsic ultrafiltration (low OCG at start of PD)	1. 機轉未明。 2. 可能跟水通道表現異常有關。	1. 避免體液容積過量。
Acquired intrinsic ultrafiltration insufficiency (low OCG developing over time years on PD)	1. 腹膜漸進性纖維化。	1. 討論造成 EPS 的可能性。 2. 轉換成其他 RRT。 3. 醫療團隊和病人一起舉行 SDM。

Abbreviations: APD, automated peritoneal dialysis; CAPD, continuous ambulatory peritoneal dialysis; EPS, encapsulating peritoneal sclerosis; OCG, osmotic conductance to glucose; PD, peritoneal dialysis; PSTR, peritoneal solute transfer rate; RRT, renal replacement therapy; SDM, shared decision-making.

```
┌─────────────────────────┐
│    Low UF Capacity      │
│ Net UF < 400 mL after   │
│ using 4.25% dextrose    │
│ solution for 4 hours    │
└─────────────────────────┘
            ↓
┌─────────────────────────┐
│ 排除 mechanical         │
│ problems/leaks          │
└─────────────────────────┘
       ↓           ↓
┌──────────────┐  ┌──────────────────┐
│ Fast Peritoneal│  │ Low Osmotic      │
│ Solute Transfer│  │ Conductance to   │
│ Rate           │  │ Glucose          │
│ Inherent       │  │ Intrinsic        │
│ Acquired       │  │ Acquired         │
│ (長期 PD／     │  │ (腹膜纖維化／    │
│  腹膜炎)       │  │  血管病變)       │
└──────────────┘  └──────────────────┘
```

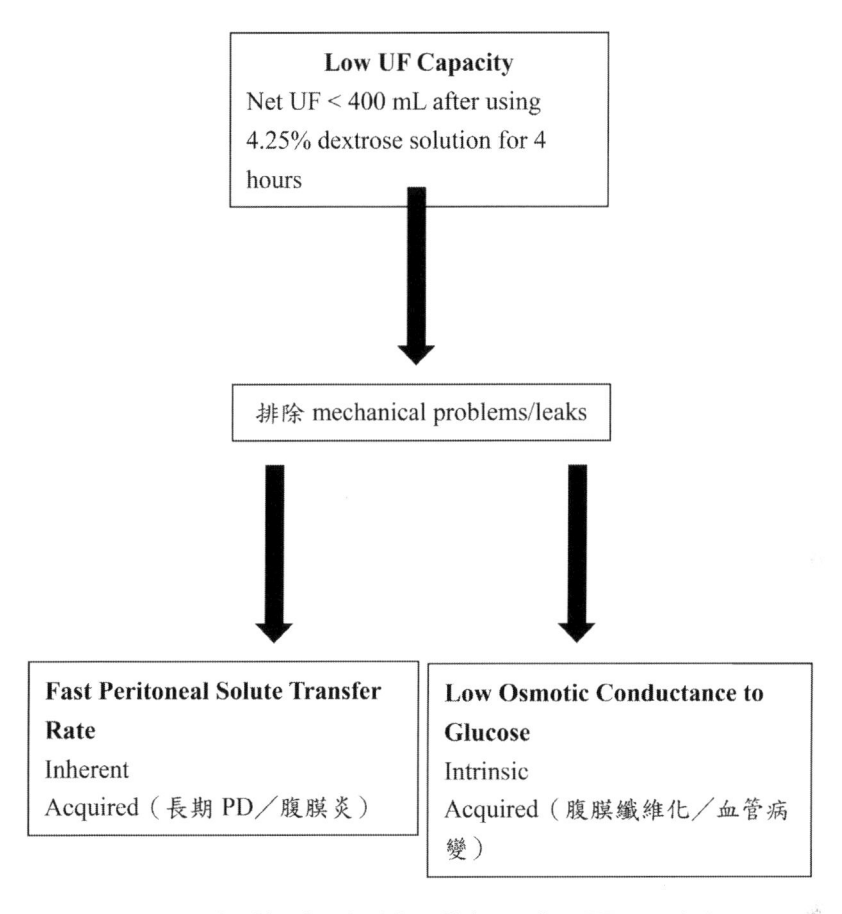

Figure 9-5. Ultrafiltration (UF) insufficiency (low UF capacity) causes

Abbreviations: PD, peritoneal dialysis.

（六）造成 UFI 的其它原因為何？

1. Mechanical problems 影響 dialysate drainage。
2. Dialysate leakage outside the peritoneal space.
3. 高 intraperitoneal pressure 導致 reversal in flow of fluid，造成逆流回 capillary bed、peritoneal tissues 或被 lymphatic absorption（Figure 9-5）[5]。

九、代謝性併發症 (Metabolic Complications)

（一）Hyperglycemia.
（二）Hyperlipidemia (triglyceride ↑, total cholesterol ↑, low-density lipoprotein cholesterol ↑, high-density lipoprotein cholesterol ↓).

（三）Protein loss (albumin) and malnutrition.

（附註：The KDOQI guidelines recommend a dietary protein intake of 1.2–1.3 g/kg/day for PD patients.）

（四）Hypokalemia.

十、感染性併發症 (Infectious Complications)

圖請參考 Figure 9-1。

（一）Peritonitis

（二）Exit-site infection

（三）Tunnel infection

十一、腹膜炎 (Peritonitis)

（一）常見的腹膜炎症狀？

最常見的三大症狀為：cloudy peritoneal fluid、abdominal pain 及 fever。

（二）Cloudy Dialysate 的鑑別診斷

詳見 Table 9-8 [5]

Table 9-8. Cloudy dialysate 的鑑別診斷 [a]

Type	Differential diagnosis
Non-cellular	1. Calcium-channel blocker.
	2. Excessive fibrin production (prolonged period of peritoneal rest).
	3. Chylous ascites.
	4. Acute pancreatitis.
Cellular	1. Infectious peritonitis.
	2. Malignancy (lymphoma, peritoneal metastasis).
	3. Allergic reaction/chemical peritonitis (eosinophilia, vancomycin, icodextrin).
	4. Menstrual-related problem.
	5. Hemoperitoneum.
	6. Specimen taken from dry abdomen (prolonged period of peritoneal rest).

[a] 參考資料來源：[5]。

（三）如何診斷腹膜炎？

至少符合兩項以下描述：1. Clinical features consistent with peritonitis, such as abdominal pain or cloudy dialysis effluent; 2. Dialysis effluent white blood cell count (WBC) > 100/mL or > 0.1×10^9/L（在腹膜內滯留至少兩小時）, with > 50% polymorphonuclear leukocytes (PMN); 3. Positive dialysis effluent culture [5].

（四）判讀 Gram Stain 結果時要注意什麼？

Gram stain preparations of PD effluent 在檢測細菌方面非常不敏感，但可早期偵測 yeast 的存在。

（五）PD 液培養要如何收集？

Peritoneal culture collection is by inoculating 5–10 mL of effluent directly into two blood culture bottle（嗜氧和厭氧）, and the sample should be sent to the laboratory within 6 hours.

（六）腹內滯留時間過短的透析液是否會干擾判讀結果？

1. 儘管有腹膜炎的臨床症狀，滯留時間過短可能會導致 low leukocyte counts。這在接受 automated peritoneal dialysis (APD) 的腎友身上更容易看到（因為滯留時間短）。故若臨床上依然高度懷疑腹膜炎，請讓透析藥水在腹內靜置兩小時後重複檢驗 cell counts 和 cultures。
2. 接受 APD 的腎友應使用 percentage of PMN 而非 absolute WBC count 來診斷腹膜炎。PMN 比例大於 50% 即可高度懷疑腹膜炎，無論 absolute WBC count 是否大於 100/mL [5]。
3. 接受 APD 的腎友若無 daytime exchange 但合併腹痛懷疑腹膜炎時，可先灌入 1 L of dialysis solution，靜置兩小時後再將引流液送檢 [5]。

（七）腹膜炎的感染途徑為何？

1. Intraluminal contamination (touch contamination).（最常見！）
2. Periluminal contamination (exit-site or tunnel infection).
3. Transvisceral migration from a bowel.
4. Vaginal leak.
5. Hematogenous dissemination from a remote source (dental procedures).

（八）Terminology for Peritonitis

詳見 Table 9-9. [5]。

（九）導致腹膜炎最常見的致病菌為何？

Majority gram-positive: *Staphylococcus epidermidis* > *Staphylococcus aureus* > *Enterococcus*.

（附註：Most common organism in fungal peritonitis: *Candida albicans*.）

（十）腹膜炎如何治療？

1. International Society of Peritoneal Dialysis (ISPD) [5] 建議 empiric therapy 要可同時治療 gram-positive 和 gram-negative 菌種。
2. 建議：vancomycin OR a first-generation cephalosporin (cefazolin) + aminoglycoside OR ceftazidime.
3. 腹膜炎病人抵達醫療機構後，抗生素每晚一小時給予，PD failure 或 death 的風險會上升 by 5.5% [5]。

（十一）腹膜炎需要治療多久？劑量為何？

1. Antibiotics course: usually 2 weeks, but *S. aureus* and *Pseudomonas*: 3 weeks.
2. Suggested intraperitoneal doses for selected antibiotics are listed in Table 9-10.

Table 9-9. Outcome specific definition following peritonitis[a]

腹膜炎之名詞	定義
Medical cure	Complete resolution of peritonitis 無合併其他以下併發症： 1. relapse/recurrent peritonitis. 2. catheter removal. 3. transfer to hemodialysis for ≥ 30 days. 4. death.
Refractory	腹膜炎在適當抗生素治療五天後透析液依然混濁。
Recurrent	腹膜炎完治後四週內復發且透析液出現不同菌種感染。
Relapsing	腹膜炎完治後四週內復發且透析液出現同一菌種感染。
Repeat	腹膜炎完治後四週後復發且透析液出現同一菌種感染。
Peritonitis-associated catheter removal	移除 PD 導管的情形為腹膜炎合併管路出口感染 (exit-site infection) 及管路通道感染 (tunnel infection)，且為同一致病菌種。

Abbreviation: PD, peritoneal dialysis.

[a] 參考資料來源：[5]。

Table 9-10. Intraperitoneal doses of selected antibiotics[a,b]

Antibiotics	Intermittent IP dose (= 1 exchange daily for at least 6 hours)
Cefazolin	15–20 mg/kg per bag once a day
Ceftazidime	15–20 mg/kg per bag once a day
Cefepime	1,000 mg per bag once a day
Gentamycin	0.6 mg/kg per bag once a day
Amikacin	2 mg/kg per bag once a day
Vancomycin	15–30 mg/kg every 5–7 days for CAPD
	15 mg/kg every 4 days for APD
Fluconazole	200 mg per bag every 24–48 hours

Abbreviations: APD, automated peritoneal dialysis; CAPD, continuous ambulatory peritoneal dialysis; IP, intraperitoneal.

[a] 參考資料來源：[5]。
[b] 建議使用 adjunctive oral N-acetylcysteine therapy 預防 aminoglycoside ototoxicity [5]。

（十二）抗生素給藥路徑該用 IP 或 Intravenous (IV)？

1. Intraperitoneal dosing 應優先被使用，但當病人 bacteremic 或 overtly septic 時，IV antibiotics 應當被優先考慮。
2. 在 dialysis effluent specimens 被收集到後，應當盡快給予抗生素，切勿因為等待檢查結果延誤抗生素治療 [5]。

（十三）IP 給藥上有哪兩種方式？

1. Intermittent administration: once a day in the longest dwell of at least 6 hours (nighttime fill for CAPD, daytime dwell for CCPD).
2. Continuous administration: dosage with each exchange.

（十四）Intermittent Administration 和 Continuous Administration 何者治療效果較佳？

Equally efficacious.

（十五）Culture-Negative Peritonitis (= Dialysate Culture Negative + Dialysate Leukocytosis) 的鑑別診斷？

1. 檢體收集程序或是實驗室處理不良。
2. 先前有使用過抗生素治療。

3. 致病菌是 fungi 或 mycobacteria。
4. Eosinophilic or chemical (e.g., icodextrin) peritonitis.

（十六）Eosinophilic Peritonitis (>10% Eosinophils in a Cloudy Effluent) 的鑑別診斷？

1. Early after catheter placement.
2. Fungal, mycotic infections.
3. Allergic reactions.
4. Exposure to drugs (vancomycin).

（十七）何謂 Enteric Peritonitis，何時該懷疑此診斷？

1. 腹膜炎起因於 enteric causes，例如：strangulated bowel、ischemic colitis 或 appendicitis 等。Morbidity 和 mortality 超過 50%。
2. 當腹膜液出現 multiple organisms (particularly both gram-positive and gram-negative) 就要高度懷疑 enteric peritonitis。
3. Enteric peritonitis 也可以 culture-negative peritonitis 表現，例如：pancreatitis [5]。

（十八）Indication for PD Catheter Removal？

詳見 Table 9-11。

（十九）低血鉀與 H_2 Receptor Antagonists 與 Peritonitis 之間的相關性？

1. 低血鉀可能會增加 peritonitis 風險。
2. Histamine-2 receptor antagonists 可能會增加 peritonitis 風險 [5]。

Table 9-11. Indications for PD catheter removal.

Indication	Clinical conditions
Absolute	1. Refractory peritonitis.
	2. Relapsing peritonitis.
	3. Fungal peritonitis[a].
Relative	1. Repeated peritonitis.
	2. Mycobacterial peritonitis.
	3. Multiple enteric organisms[b].

[a] 拔管後抗生素還要持續使用 10 天。
[b] 需考慮做腹部影像檢查和外科介入治療。

（二十）腹膜炎的病人皆需照 Abdominal X-ray？

Abdominal X-ray 並非腹膜炎的常規檢查，且 abdominal X-ray 常會顯示 pneumoperitoneum（約 1/3 的 CAPD 腎友，因換液時空氣會從 PD tube 進入腹膜）導致誤判為 perforated peptic ulcer [5]。

（二十一）腹膜炎的病人是否需做 Peripheral Blood Cultures？

1. Peripheral blood cultures 一般結果都是陰性，故除非病人臨床上顯示 septic 或 immunosuppression，不須常規檢測 [5]。
2. 當培養顯示 bacteremia，要高度懷疑腹內有其他病灶的可能性。

十二、管路出口感染 (Exit-Site Infection) 及管路通道感染 (Tunnel Infection)

（一）Exit-Site Infections 的常見臨床表現為何？

1. 導管皮膚交界處出現 swelling。
2. 導管皮膚交界處出現 crust。
3. 導管皮膚交界處出現 redness。
4. 導管皮膚交界處出現 pain 或 pressure。
5. 導管皮膚交界處出現 secretion (purulent discharge)。

（附註：Crust formation 出現在 exit-site 不一定就是感染。Positive wound cultures 倘若無其他相關症狀可能僅是 colonization。）

（二）Tunnel Infection 的臨床表現為何？

The presence of inflammation (erythema, edema, tenderness, or induration) along the tunnel.

（三）管路出口感染和管路通道感染最常見的致病菌為何？

S. aureus.

（四）管路出口感染和管路通道感染應如何治療？

詳見 Table 9-12。

Table 9-12. Treatment strategy for Gram (+) and Gram (−) organisms

類別	治療
Gram (+)	Gram-positive organisms can be treated with an oral cephalosporin or penicillinase-resistant antibiotic. Resistant strains may require vancomycin.
Gram (−)	Gram-negative organisms can usually be treated with oral ciprofloxacin (500 mg bid); with *Pseudomonas aeruginosa*, addition of ceftazidime or an aminoglycoside may become necessary, as well as catheter removal.

（五）管路出口感染和管路通道感染需治療多久？

　　Antibiotics course: usually 2 weeks, but Pseudomonas: 3 weeks.

（六）何時需考慮拔除 PD 導管？

1. Refractory peritonitis.
2. Relapsing peritonitis.
3. Patients whose exit-site or tunnel infection progresses to peritonitis.
4. Fungal peritonitis.

（七）是否有藥物可減少 PD 導管感染的機會？

　　每日在 exit-site 塗抹 0.1% gentamicin cream 可減少 exit-site infections (*S. aureus* 和 *Pseudomonas aeruginosa*)。

十三、機械性併發症 (Mechanical Complications)

（一）Impaired dialysate flow，可能原因如下：

1. Constipation.
2. Catheter migration.
3. Kinking of the catheter.
4. Adhesion formation.
5. Omental wrapping.
6. Fibrin plugging.

（二）Back pain.

（三）Hernias (10%–20% of PD patients).

（四）Pericatheter leakage (abdominal/genital edema).

（五）Diaphragmatic leakage (hydrothorax).（一般都在右側肋膜）
　　（附註：A diagnostic thoracentesis reveals markedly elevated glucose levels when the pleural fluid originates from the peritoneal solution.）
（六）Sclerosing encapsulating peritonitis.

十四、包囊性腹膜硬化症 (Sclerosing Encapsulating Peritonitis)

（一）Sclerosing encapsulating peritonitis 是因腹膜 fibrous transformation 導致 bowel loops entraps，造成 intestinal obstruction、nausea、vomiting 和 anorexia。
（二）當出現 bloody dialysis fluid 時應將包囊性腹膜硬化症列入鑑別診斷。
（三）發病率約 2.5%，在 long-term PD (> 5–8 years) 的腎友身上更容易看到。
（四）腹部 computed tomography 可能看到的影像表現為何？
1. Peritoneal thickening and calcification.
2. Bowel thickening, tethering, dilatation, obstruction.
3. Loculated ascites.
（五）應如何治療？
1. Discontinuation of PD.
2. Bowel rest.
3. Nutritional support.
4. Surgical lysis of adhesions when obstruction occurs.
5. Immunosuppression with prednisone (10–40 mg/day) (modest benefit).
6. Tamoxifen (20 mg bid) (in case series).
（六）預後如何？
　　Poor (with a 1-year mortality rate > 50%).

十五、PD 何時該轉換成血液透析？

（一）Common Reasons for a Permanent Switch Include the Following

1. 無法達足量透析 (Kt/V_{urea} < 1.7)。
2. 脫水量不足 (UF failure)。
3. 無法以藥物治療的 severe hypertriglyceridemia。
4. 頻繁的發生腹膜炎。

5. 無法以手術治療的機械性問題 (sclerosis encapsulating peritonitis)。
6. Severe protein malnutrition resistant to aggressive management.

（二）Common Reasons for a Temporary Switch Include the Following

1. 手術有觸及腹膜腔（perforated ulcer 或 bowel obstruction 等）。
2. 腹膜液滲漏。
3. 感染併發症需暫時移除 PD tube。

參考文獻

[1] Ellsworth PI. Peritoneal dialysis catheter insertion. Medscape Website. https://emedicine.medscape.com/article/1829737-overview. Accessed April, 29, 2023

[2] Taal MW, Chertow GM, Marsden PA, Skorecki K, Yu ASL, Brenner BM, eds. *Brenner and Rector's The Kidney*. 9th ed. Philadelphia, PA: Elsevier; 2011.

[3] Baxter Healthcare Corporation. GlucoseSafety. Baxter Healthcare Corporation Web site. https://www.glucosesafety.com/index.html. Accessed April, 29, 2023

[4] Karl ZJT, Khanna ONR, Leonor BFP, Ryan P, Moore HL, Nielsen MP. Peritoneal equilibration test. *Perit Dial Int*. 1987;7(3):138-148. doi:10.1177/089686088700700306

[5] Li PKT, Chow KM, Cho Y, et al. ISPD peritonitis guideline recommendations: 2022 update on prevention and treatment [published correction appears in Perit Dial Int. 2023;8968608231166870]. *Perit Dial Int*. 2022;42(2):110-153. doi:10.1177/08968608221080586

延伸閱讀文獻

Bernardini J, Bender F, Florio T, et al. Randomized, double-blind trial of antibiotic exit site cream for prevention of exit site infection in peritoneal dialysis patients. *J Am Soc Nephrol*. 2005;16(2):539-545. doi:10.1681/ASN.2004090773

Brown EA, Davies SJ, Rutherford P, et al. Survival of functionally anuric patients on automated peritoneal dialysis: the European APD Outcome Study. *J Am Soc Nephrol*. 2003;14(11):2948-2957. doi:10.1097/01.asn.0000092146.67909.e2

Churchill DN, Thorpe KE, Nolph KD, Keshaviah PR, Oreopoulos DG, Pagé D. Increased peritoneal membrane transport is associated with decreased patient and technique survival for continuous peritoneal dialysis patients. The Canada-USA (CANUSA) Peritoneal Dialysis Study Group. *J Am Soc Nephrol*. 1998;9(7):1285-1292. doi:10.1681/ASN.V971285

Ellsworth PI. Peritoneal dialysis catheter insertion. Medscape Website. https://emedicine.medscape.

com/article/1829737-overview.

Karl ZJT, Khanna ONR, Leonor BFP, Ryan P, Moore HL, Nielseb MP. Peritoneal equilibration test. *Perit Dial Int*. 1987;7(3):138-148. doi:10.1177/089686088700700306

Li PKT, Chow KM, Cho Y, et al. ISPD peritonitis guideline recommendations: 2022 update on prevention and treatment [published correction appears in *Perit Dial Int*. 2023;8968608231166870]. *Perit Dial Int*. 2022;42(2):110-153. doi:10.1177/08968608221080586

Li PK, Szeto CC, Piraino B, et al. ISPD peritonitis recommendations: 2016 update on prevention and treatment [published correction appears in *Perit Dial Int*. 2018;38(4):313]. *Perit Dial Int*. 2016;36(5):481-508. doi:10.3747/pdi.2016.00078

Lo WK, Ho YW, Li CS, et al. Effect of Kt/V on survival and clinical outcome in CAPD patients in a randomized prospective study. *Kidney Int*. 2003;64(2):649-656. doi:10.1046/j.1523-1755.2003.00098.x

Mehrotra R, Ravel V, Streja E, et al. Peritoneal equilibration test and patient outcomes. *Clin J Am Soc Nephrol*. 2015;10(11):1990-2001. doi:10.2215/CJN.03470315

Moncrief JW, Popovich RP, Nolph KD. The history and current status of continuous ambulatory peritoneal dialysis. *Am J Kidney Dis*. 1990;16(6):579-584. doi:10.1016/s0272-6386(12)81044-4

Morelle J, Stachowska-Pietka J, Öberg C, et al. ISPD recommendations for the evaluation of peritoneal membrane dysfunction in adults: classification, measurement, interpretation and rationale for intervention. *Perit Dial Int*. 2021;41(4):352-372. doi:10.1177/0896860820982218

Paniagua R, Amato D, Vonesh E, et al. Effects of increased peritoneal clearances on mortality rates in peritoneal dialysis: ADEMEX, a prospective, randomized, controlled trial. *J Am Soc Nephrol*. 2002;13(5):1307-1320. doi:10.1681/ASN.V1351307

Taal MW, Chertow GM, Marsden PA, Skorecki K, Yu ASL, Brenner BM, eds. *Brenner and Rector's the Kidney*. 9th ed. Philadelphia, PA: Elsevier; 2011.

Chapter 10

Common Problems in Patients with Renal Transplant

楊晴涵
皇秦診所

吳采虹
臺北榮民總醫院腎臟科

一、Introduction

自 1954 年全球第一次成功的腎臟移植以來,已經有超過 500,000 個 end-stage renal disease 病患受惠於腎臟移植。依臺灣健保資料分析證實腎臟移植病人的五年存活率遠高於透析治療 (93% vs. 56%),其中活體捐贈的長期存活率又優於屍腎移植,但相較於透析病患皆有更好的生活品質。所以腎臟移植對 chronic kidney disease (CKD) 病患 (glomerular filtration rate [GFR] < 20 mL/min) 來說是較好的腎臟替代療法的選擇。

二、Patient Selection

(一) Recipient Evaluation

腎臟移植的禁忌症很少,大多是相對禁忌症而非絕對禁忌症。除了 Table 10-1 的禁忌症外,age/obesity/prior kidney transplantation/underlying renal diseases 也是要特別注意的部分。

1. Age

以下兩個年齡層跟其他年齡層比較起來 graft survival 比較差:(1) Adolescent patients (age 12–17) 和 (2) Elderly patients (age > 65)。推測是因為這群病患遵醫囑性較差及高齡的病人免疫抑制劑的併發症較多或死於非移植相關併發症風險較高的緣故。

Table 10-1. Contraindications to transplantation

Contraindication	Clinical conditions
Absolute	Active infection
	Disseminated malignancy
	Extensive vascular disease
	High risk for perioperative mortality
	Persistent coagulation abnormality
	Informed patient refusal of consent
Relative	Renal disease with high recurrence rate
	Urologic abnormalities
	Active systemic illness
	Ongoing substances abuse
	Uncontrolled psychosis
	Refractory nonadherence

2. Obesity

肥胖不是移植的絕對禁忌症，但的確是一個重要的危險因子。Body mass index (BMI) > 35 kg/m^2 和 poor post-transplant prognosis 相關。

3. Prior Kidney Transplantation

要接受二次移植的病患應詳細檢討可能導致 graft failure 的原因，包括：non-adherence with immunosuppressive medications、recurrent renal disease 或 high allo-reactivity with high panel reactive antibody (PRA) titers 等等。

4. Underlying Renal Diseases

主要透過三方面影響腎臟移植後的結果：
(1) Etiologic mechanism.
(2) Propensity of recurrence.
(3) Status of immune system.

（二）Organ Donors

腎臟來源不夠一直是腎臟移植的瓶頸，統計顯示臺灣於 2021 年等待腎臟移植人數超過七千人，一年大體腎臟捐贈移植數卻僅有一百多例，親屬間活體腎臟捐贈移植人數雖有逐年增加，但仍有多數人苦等移植機會。原按照《人體器官移植條例》的規定，受移植者必須是捐贈者五等親以內之血親或配偶，為增加等待換腎病人成功接受移植的機會，臺灣衛生福利部於 2019 年通過非親屬間的活腎交換移植手術，明定合適腎臟捐贈者得以在自主意願下，經器官移植醫學倫理委員會審查通過，可進行交換捐贈移植手術。

1. Living Donors

Living related donors 和 living unrelated donors 腎臟移植的預後相近，都比 deceased donors 的預後來得好。Table 10-2 為 living donor 的 exclusion criteria。

2. Deceased Donors

過去因待捐贈者數量遠超過腦死捐贈 (donation after brain death, DBD) 者，促使全世界開始發展活體捐贈與心臟循環停止後的器官捐贈 (donation after circulatory death, DCD)。

(1) DBD
　　A. Standard criteria donors：小於 60 歲的健康成人。

Table 10-2. Exclusion criteria for living kidney donors[a]

Age < 18 or > 65–70	Acute symptomatic infection
Bilateral, recurrent kidney stones	Uncontrolled psychiatric illness
Active cancer or incompletely treated cancer	Uncontrolled hypertension or with evidence of end-organ damage
Proteinuria (> 300 mg/day)	Microscopic hematuria
Abnormal GFR (< 60 mL/min)	Type 1 diabetes mellitus

Abbreviation: GFR, glomerular filtration rate.
[a]Urologic/vascular abnormalities in donor kidneys.

B. Expanded criteria donors： a. 大於 60 歲的健康成人。b. 50–59 歲的不健康成人，下列三項健康問題至少有兩項：Cerebrovascular accident as a cause of death; prior diagnosis of hypertension; terminal serum creatinine greater than 1.5 mg/dL。

(2) DCD

指心臟停止跳動、全身循環停止五分鐘後，才可開始進行器官捐贈。可再分為嚴密觀察控制下 (controlled) 發生的，例如在醫院內撤除維生系統後的心跳停止，與無法監測控管下 (uncontrolled) 發生的，例如醫院外急救無效、到院前心跳停止。目前臺灣推行的 DCD 捐贈模式為 controlled DCD，且不得為保存器官功能而預先置入葉克膜體外循環系統，故手術流程上更是分秒必爭，目標將溫缺血的傷害降到最低。

（三）Predictors of Outcome

1. Recipient factors: younger, low levels of PRA, have spent less time on dialysis, transplanted preemptively, nonblack, and non-Hispanic recipients.
2. Donor factors: living donors, younger age, shorter cold ischemia time, and nonblack donors.
3. Donor/recipient compatibility: better human leukocyte antigen (HLA) matching, cytomegalovirus (CMV) serologic status matching, and equivalent donor/recipient BMI.

三、Immunology and Pharmacotherapy

（一）Immunology

Recipients 對於 allograft 的免疫反應主要透過主要組織相容複合物 (major histocompatibility complex, MHC)、antigen-presenting cells (APCs)、T cells and B cells 來完成。細胞之間的活化主要經由以下三種 signal pathways，也是免疫抑制劑作用的位置。

1. Signal 1

APC 透過 MHC 和 T cells 上的 T-cell receptor (TCR)/cluster of differentiation (CD)3 complex 結合，透過 Ca-dependent pathway 而造成 calcineurin 的活化。

2. Signal 2

又稱為 costimulatory signals，活化 T cell 單靠 signal 1 是不夠的，還需要其他 costimulatory signals，譬如 APC 上的 CD80/86 和 T cell 上的 CD28 結合，會造成後續 interleukin 2 (IL-2) 的製造及 T cell 的活化。

3. Signal 3

IL-2 結合 T cell 上的 receptor 會進一步造成後續 T cell 內的 cell cycle and proliferation。免疫反應機轉圖可參考 [1]。

（二）Pharmacotherapy

以下介紹較常使用的免疫抑制藥物。

1. The Calcineurin Inhibitors (CNIs)

Cyclosporine (CsA) 與 tacrolimus (TAC) 會分別和兩種 immunophilin protein 結合，進而阻斷 Ca-dependent antigen triggered T cell activation 而抑制免疫。共同副作用為 CNI nephrotoxicity，其他常見的副作用如 Table 10-3。值得注意的是 CsA 與 TAC 皆是透過細胞色素 P450 3A4 酶 (cytochrome P450 3A4, CYP3A4) 來代謝，故若與其他會影響 CYP3A4 活性的藥物併用時，會間接影響移植藥物的血中濃度。常見的藥物交互作用列在 Table 10-4。

2. The Mammalian Target of Rapamycin (mTOR) Inhibitors

包括 sirolimus 與 everolimus，主要透過抑制 mTOR pathway 及 CD28-mediated costimulation 路徑來抑制免疫。藥物副作用包括：aphthous stomatitis、dyslipidemia、thrombocytopenia、delayed wound healing、proteinuria、interstitial pneumonitis 等。

Table 10-3. Adverse drug effects of calcineurin inhibitors

出現頻率	副作用
CsA > TAC	Hypertrichosis, gingival hypertrophy, hyperuricemia hyperlipidemia, hypertension
TAC > CsA	Posttransplant diabetes, alopecia, hypertrophic cardiomyopathy (children), neurotoxicity

Abbreviations: CsA, cyclosporine; TAC, tacrolimus.

Table 10-4. Drug interactions with cyclosporine and tacrolimus

Class of drug	Increase CNI level	Decrease CNI level
Calcium channel blocker	Diltiazem, verapamil	—
Antibiotic	Macrolides	Nafcillin
Antifungal	Fluconazole, voriconazole	—
Antituberculous	—	Rifampin, rifabutin, isoniazid
Antiviral	Ritonavir, nelfinavir, saquinavir	Efavirenz, nevirapine
Anticonvulant	—	Phenytoin, phenobarbital, carbamazepine, primidone
Antidepressant	Fluoxetine, nefazodone, fluvoxamine	—
Food	Grapefruit juice	—
Herb	—	St. John's wort

Abbreviation: CNI, calcineurin inhibitor.

3. Azathioprine

口服吸收到體內會被轉變成 purine analog，成為 nonspecific inhibitor of purine biosynthesis，是一個 antiproliferative agent，副作用包括 cytopenia、diarrhea、hepatic dysfunction and increased risk of malignancy。勿與 allopurinol 併用，因 allopurinol 會抑制 azathioprine 的代謝，造成累積而產生相關毒性反應如嚴重骨髓抑制。

4. Mycophenolate Mofetil (MMF)

MMF 會去抑制 guanosine 的 de novo 合成所必須的 inosine monophosphate dehydrogenase，進而抑制 cell 的 proliferation。副作用包括 neutropenia and gastrointestinal side effects。

5. Corticosteroid

會抑制 T cell proliferation、T cell-dependent immunity 以及 cytokine gene transcription（IL-1、IL-2、IL-6 等等）。副作用包括 fluid and salt retention、steroid-induced diabetes、steroid psychosis、poor wound healing、increased frequency of infection、proximal myopathy、osteoporosis and osteonecrosis 等等。

6. Muromonab-CD3

是一種老鼠的單株抗體，會去攻擊 TCR 的 CD3 部分，目前是作為 induction therapy，其最惡名昭彰的副作用為 first drug reaction，主要是因為 cytokine release。

7. Antithymocyte Globulin

為多株抗體，可以用來當作 induction therapy，也可以用來治療 rejection。

8. IL-2 Receptor Antagonists

包括 basiliximab 與 daclizumab，會跟活化的 T cell 細胞膜上的 CD25 結合，競爭型的抑制 IL-2，達到抑制 allograft rejection 的目的。目前主要用作腎臟移植後的 induction therapy 使用。

9. Anti-CD20 Monoclonal Antibody (Rituximab)

為一種 CD20 的單株抗體，與 B cell 上的 CD20 抗原結合後引起免疫反應促使 B cell lysis。常與免疫球蛋白 intravenous immunoglobulin 併用在移植前 desensitization 或 acute or chronic antibody mediated rejection。

（三）加強的免疫抑制

可能是用在 induction therapy 或出現急性排斥時使用的 antirejection 治療。

（四）持續的免疫抑制

Maintenance immunosuppression 主要目的是使用持續性的免疫抑制藥物達到預防排斥的目的。傳統上會使用 2-3 種藥物治療，多管齊下阻斷 T cell 活化，包括以下不同機制：

1. Inhibitors of transcription (the CNIs).
2. Inhibitors of nucleotide synthesis (azathioprine and MMF).
3. Inhibitors of growth factor signal transduction (the mTOR inhibitors).
4. Broad immunosuppressant with inhibitory activity against lymphocytes, macrophages, and neutrophils (oral corticosteroid):
    (1) 現行標準的治療為 CNIs + anti-proliferative or mTOR inhibitors + steroid。
    (2) 因為 steroid 的諸多副作用，因此 steroid avoidance or steroid withdrawal 越來越流行，臨床試驗發現，雖然可以降低 bone disease、cataract 和 hypertriglyceridemia 的比率，但是急性排斥甚至慢性排斥的比率皆比使用 chronic standard steroid 的病患來的高，所以要拿掉 steroid 之前還是要三思。

四、Assessing Compatibility and Immunological Risk

人類白血球抗原 (HLA) 為人類的 MHC，位於第六對染色體的短臂上 (6p21.31)，是個體細胞獨一無二的組織抗原。Donor 的組織抗原對 recipient 來說是外來物，會引起 recipient 的免疫反應。HLA 分為兩型，Class I 有 HLA-A、B、C 表現在所有有核細胞的表面；Class II 有 HLA-DR、DP、DQ 表現在 B cell 及 APC 上。某些人體內原本即存在抗 HLA 抗體，高危險族群像是懷孕、常接受輸血或曾經接受移植者。HLA 抗體的偵測可作為預測排斥反應與藥物治療效果的參數之一，受贈者需要接受的排斥風險評估如下：

（一）HLA matching：HLA-A + B + HLA-DR 的 6 個抗原對偶基因配對程度與腎臟移植病患存活率相關，完全相合的移植病患存活率會高於完全不合的病患，但即使 HLA 完全不合的腎移植病患也比待移植的病人死亡風險低，故 HLA 配對不合並非移植的禁忌症。目前在腦死後捐腎者出現時可藉由 HLA 配對挑選排斥風險較低的受腎者。

（二）Crossmatch：交叉配對試驗是器官移植前最重要的檢驗項目，是以 recipient 的血清與 donor 淋巴球做補體淋巴球細胞毒性測試，可分為 T 及 B 細胞測試。若交叉配對試驗陽性之病患，表示體內具有抗此捐贈者的 HLA 抗體，移植後有很高機率產生超急性排斥，故不適合接受該捐贈者之器官。

（三）PRA：群體反應性抗體是將 recipient 的血清與當地一般族群常見的 HLA 作反應，PRA 陽性百分比代表病患體中 HLA 抗體的特異性廣泛度（而非抗體量），若百分比越高則對越多的 HLA 抗原有反應，接受移植後產生排斥的機率也越大。

（四）Donor-specific anti-HLA antibody：利用 Luminex single antigen bead anti-HLA antibody assay 可直接精準檢驗出 recipient 血清中已經存在的 donor specific 的 HLA 抗體量，但目前健保尚未給付，需自費檢驗。

五、Common Post-Transplant Complication

（一）Wound Complication

傷口相關併發症包含表皮傷口裂開 (dehiscence)、筋膜 (fascia) 裂開、傷口感染與移植腎周圍積液等。術後使用 sirolimus/everolimus 的病人較易有傷口癒合不良。

（二）Bleeding

移植術後出血常見於血管吻合處，常需手術探查以止血。

（三）Arterial Thrombosis

腎臟動脈的栓塞是很罕見的情況，發生率 < 1%，原因可能和血流灌注衝擊、貧血和尿毒症導致的凝血功能缺陷有關。

（四）Venous Thrombosis

移植腎的 renal vein thrombosis 不常見，且通常是手術時血管接得不盡理想所致，形成的因素包括 CsA 使用導致 platelet aggregation，形成 hypercoagulable status，或者因為把腎臟種到原本的 retroperitoneal space，使原本的空間組織 fibrosis 變得又硬又緊而擠壓到腎臟和血管。臨床症狀包括蛋白尿和腎臟腫大，但也可能無明顯症狀。診斷可使用 doppler plethysmography 或 venography，venography 是最好的診斷工具。

（五）Urine Leak

Urine leak 是個不常見但很嚴重的併發症，發生率大約是 2%，漏尿的地方可能是 renal calyx、ureter 與 bladder。由於 urine 對組織來說是一種很強的 chemical irritant，且會使剛接好的 vascular anastomosis 的感染風險大增。臨床症狀在一開始時不太明顯，常常要等到積一大包尿在肚子裡產生感染才會被發現。

（六）Ureteral Obstruction

可分成 acute ureteral obstruction 與 remote ureteral obstruction。

1. Acute Ureteral Obstruction
(1) 可能是 distal ureter 的 ischemia/infarction/rejection 所導致。也有可能是 blood clot 卡住，若是 ureter/bladder blood clot 導致尿路阻塞通常 3-way Foley normal saline irrigation 可解決。
(2) 手術導致輸尿管進到膀胱處阻塞的情形很少見，若不幸發生，臨床上會在腎臟移植手術後「立即」發生寡尿／無尿現象。

2. Remote Ureteral Obstruction
病生理機轉：Chronic ischemia→ fibrosis→ stricture→ progressive azotemia over months。（所以腎臟移植病患腎功能逐漸惡化一定要想到有此可能的 post-renal 原因導致 acute kidney injury on CKD）

（七）Lymphocele

臨床上常常沒有特別的症狀，但也可能因為擠壓到周邊的組織而產生症狀，診斷可使用 ultrasonography。Lymphocele 裡的 lymph 是從 recipient iliac vessels 的淋巴管來，而非來自 graft kidney 的 renal hilum。所以最好的預防策略就是在腎臟移植手術時把淋巴管確實結紮。

六、Renal Complication

（一）Delayed Graft Function (DGF)

DGF 的定義是在移植後一週內（腎功能還未恢復）需要接受透析。最常見的原因是 post-ischemic acute tubular necrosis，而造成的因素通常是 donor hypovolemia/hypotension 或是 prolonged cold、warm ischemia during recovery、preservation。當病人一旦發生 DGF 時，要先安排超音波排除 technical causes，且要考慮何時做腎臟切片以排除排斥反應造成的 DGF。

（二）Rejection

Rejection 是最主要造成 graft failure 的原因之一，因此最好能及早診斷急性排斥，然後根據其病理分類儘早對症下藥。

1. Hyperacute Antibody-Mediated Rejection (AMR)

Hyperacute AMR 通常都是因為有 preformed antibodies，通常都是在手術 perfusion 時發生，而造成 immediate graft dysfunction。

2. Acute T Cell-Mediated (Cellular) Rejection

可以在移植後任何時間發生，但最常發生的時間落在移植後的 1–4 週。在過往免疫抑制劑較不發達的時代臨床症狀較明顯，包括腎臟腫脹疼痛、oliguria、腎功能惡化及發燒等症狀，但現在免疫抑制劑進步，臨床症狀較不明顯。所以常常須要借助腎臟切片協助鑑別診斷。

3. Acute Antibody-Mediated Rejection

可能在移植後的任何時間單獨出現或者合併 acute cellular rejection。診斷的 triad 包括：(1) tissue injury (classically, peritubular capillaritis composed primarily of neutrophils),

(2) the presence of circulating anti-donor antibodies (donor specific antibodies), (3) evidence of complement activation via staining for C4d。上述三個條件都成立可以達成特異性高的 acute AMR 診斷。

（三）Recurrent Disease

嚴格來說，所有的腎絲球腎炎在腎臟移植後都有可能會復發，只是復發頻率、臨床表現和預後各不相同罷了！臨床表現的症狀包括：proteinuria、microscopic、hematuria、nephrotic syndrome 以及 loss of function。

（四）Chronic Allograft Nephropathy

Chronic allograft nephropathy 是一個 non-specific syndrome，主要的臨床表現是 progressive kidney failure、proteinuria 以及 hypertension。主要造成的原因分成 immunologic and non-immunologic factors：

1. Immunologic Factors
(1) Episodes of acute rejection: poor HLA matching and previous sensitization, DGF.
(2) Subacute and chronic alloimmune response: suboptimal immunosuppression, noncompliance of patient.

2. Non-Immunologic Factors
(1) Acute peri-transplantational injuries: brain-death injury, preservation injury, or ischemic injury.
(2) Older donor or poor graft quality.
(3) Hypertension, hyperlipidemia.
(4) Chronic toxic effects of CNIs.

七、Medical Complications

（一）Infectious Disease

腎臟移植病患的感染主要受兩大因素交互影響：(1) immunosuppression 程度； (2) epidemiologic exposures。感染的症狀最主要就是發燒，Table 10-5 提供了一個移植病患發燒診斷流程供參考。移植後的第一個月很少發生伺機性感染，此時的感染併發風險症和一般泌尿道大手術類似。移植後的第 1-6 個月則因為免疫抑制藥物的藥效最強，

Table 10-5. The diagnosis approach to the transplant patient with an unexplained fever

Possible site of infection	Investigations
• Chest: pulmonary infection, pericarditis, endocarditis • Mouth: candida • Lower limb: DVT • Soft tissue: skin, joints • Transplant wound: rejection, abscess, urine leak • Peritoneal cavity: pancreas, colon, dialysis catheter • Urinary tract: bladder, prostate • CNS: *Listeria, Cryptococcus, Aspergillus* • Systemic: viral infection, tuberculosis	• CXR • Ultrasound of transplanted kidney • Cultures: mouth, sputum, urine, blood, stool, access sites • Serology: viral antibodies, especially CMV • Lumbar puncture and CT of head if CNS infection suspected

Abbreviations: CMV, cytomegalovirus; CNS, central nervous system; CT, computed tomography; CXR, chest X-ray; DVT, deep vein thrombosis.

且同時可能因為發生排斥而必須使用強力抗排斥藥物，所以免疫低下而容易有伺機性感染，包括：*Cryptococcus*、*Candida*、*Aspergillus*、*Pneumocystis jirovecii*、CMV 以及 herpes zoster。

（二）Cardiovascular Disease (CVD)

CVD 是腎臟移植病患 mortality and morbidity 最主要的原因之一，風險因子包括：underlying disease for renal failure (e.g., diabetes)、CKD 本身就是 CVD 的風險因子、tobacco use、diabetes、obesity、hypertension 和 dyslipidemia 等等。

（三）Malignancy

移植病患在移植後癌症的發生率因地而異，歐洲約 1.6%，澳洲約 24%。最常見的癌症是 skin cancer 和 malignant lymphoma，撇開這兩種癌症不談，其他各種癌症發生的機率在移植後都顯著上升（詳見 Table 10-6）。腎臟移植患者罹癌風險增加的機轉如下：

1. Depression of immune surveillance.
2. Chronic antigenic stimulation in the presence of immunosuppression.
3. Directly neoplastic action of the immunosuppressive drugs themselves.
4. Increased susceptibility to oncogenic viral infection.
    (1) Papilloma virus → squamous cell carcinoma antigen, condyloma acuminatum, cervical cancer.
    (2) Epstein-Barr virus → polyclonal B cell lymphoproliferative disease.

Table 10-6. Common malignancies encountered in renal transplant recipients

Cancer	Increased risk compared to general population
Cancer of the skin and lips	> 20×
Squamous cell carcinoma	
Basal cell carcinoma	
Malignant melanoma	
Malignant lymphoma	> 20×
Non-Hodgkin lymphoma	
Reticulum cell sarcoma	
B-cell lymphoproliferative syndrome	
Kaposi sarcoma	> 20×
Cutaneous form	
Visceral and cutaneous form	
Genitourinary cancer	> 15×
Carcinoma of native kidney	
Carcinoma of transplanted kidney	
Carcinoma of the urinary bladder	
Uroepithelial tumors	
Gynecologic cancer	5×
Carcinoma of cervix	
Ovarian cancer	

（四）Bone Disease

Renal osteodystrophy 最常見是 secondary hyperparathyroidism 和 osteomalacia。而成功的腎臟移植，會因為鈣磷代謝及酸血症的校正而有助於骨病變的改善。但是腎臟移植後 corticosteroids 和 CNIs 的使用卻會導致 osteoporosis 移植後的前 6 個月因為 steroid 還無法減量，所以骨質流失速度最快。腎臟移植病患發生 atraumatic fractures 的盛行率高達 22%，主要發生在 high cancellous bone 像是 vertebrae 和 ribs。腎臟移植病患的骨病變處理十分複雜，建議用 dual energy X-ray absorptiometry 定期追蹤 lumbar spine and hip-bone mineral densities (time of transplant, after 6 months, and then every 12 months if results are abnormal.)。如果一開始骨密度就很低或者骨質流失很快的病患，建議可以補鈣（1g/d，如果病患沒有高鈣血症的話），給予 Vitamin D 補充 (e.g., calcitriol)，也可以考慮使用 calcitonin 和 bisphosphonate。

參考文獻

[1] Halloran PF. Immunosuppressive drugs for kidney transplantation [published correction appears in *N Engl J Med*. 2005;352(10):1056]. *N Engl J Med*. 2004;351(26):2715-2729. doi:10.1056/NEJMra033540

延伸閱讀文獻

Gibney E, Parikh C, Jani A. The patient with a kidney transplant. In: Schrier RW, ed. *Manual of Nephrology*. 7th ed. Philadelphia, PA: Lippincott Williams and Wilkins;2009:204-219.

Halloran PF. Immunosuppressive drugs for kidney transplantation [published correction appears in *N Engl J Med*. 2005;352(10):1056]. *New Engl J Med*. 2004;351(26):2715-2729. doi:10.1056/NEJMra033540

Taiwan Organ Registry and Sharing Center. Origins Website. https://www.torsc.org.tw/about/about_08.jsp

Wiseman AC, Cooper JE, Chan L. Clinical aspects of renal transplantation. In: Schrier RW, Coffman TM, Falk RJ, Molitoris BA, Neilson EG, eds. *Schrier's Diseases of the Kidney*. 9th ed. Philadelphia, PA: Wolters Kluwer Health; 2012:2380-2437.

Yu ASL, Chertow GM, Luyckx VA, Marsden PA, Skorecki K, Taal MW, eds. *Brenner and Rector's The Kidney*. 11th ed. Philadelphia, PA: Elsevier; 2019.

Chapter 11

Common Problems in Patients with Acute Kidney Injury

何揚
臺北榮民總醫院腎臟科
李國華
臺北榮民總醫院腎臟科
唐德成
臺北榮民總醫院腎臟科

I. How to Define Acute Kidney Injury (AKI)?

(I) Definition

Rapid (hours to days) decline in glomerular filtration rate (GFR) and/or reduction of urine output (Table 11-1).

A. Serum Creatinine

An increase in serum creatinine $\geq$ 0.3 mg/dL over < 48 hrs or an increase of $\geq$ 50% over < 7 days.

B. Urine Output < 0.5 mL/kg/h for > 6 hrs
(A) Non-oliguric AKI: daily U/O > 400 mL.
(B) Oliguric AKI: daily U/O < 400 mL.
(C) Anuric AKI: daily U/O < 100 mL.

(II) Acute Kidney Disease

AKI or a reduction in the GFR to less than 60 mL/min/1.73 m^2 a decrease in the GFR by 35% or more, an increase in the serum creatinine level by more than 50%, or the presence of structural kidney damage of less than 3 months' duration.

(III) Operational Definition and Staging Criteria of AKI: RIFLE (Risk, Injury, Failure, Loss of Kidney Function, and End-Stage Kidney Disease), AKIN (Acute Kidney Injury Network), and KDIGO (Kidney Disease: Improving Global Outcomes)

II. What Are AKI Risk Factors?

(I) Clinical History

A. Elderly.
B. Chronic kidney disease (CKD).
C. Diabetes mellitus (DM).

Table 11-1. Definition and staging of acute kidney injury

Definitions

	RIFLE	AKIN	KDIGO
SCr	An increase of ≥ 50% developing over < 7 days	An increase of ≥ 0.3 mg/dL or of ≥ 50% developing over < 48 hrs	An increase of ≥ 0.3 mg/dL developing over < 48 hrs or an increase of ≥ 50% developing over < 7 days
Urine output[a]	< 0.5 mL/kg/h for > 6 hrs		

Staging criteria

RIFLE	SCr increase	AKIN	SCr increase	KDIGO	SCr increase	Urine output[a]
Risk	≥ 50%	Stage 1	≥ 0.3 mg/dL or ≥ 50%	Stage 1	≥ 0.3 mg/dL or ≥ 50%	< 0.5 mL/kg/h for > 6 hrs
Injury	≥ 100%	Stage 2	≥ 100%	Stage 2	≥ 100%	< 0.5 mL/kg/h for > 12 hrs
Failure	≥ 200%	Stage 3	≥ 200%	Stage 3	≥ 200%	< 0.3 mL/kg/h for > 24 hrs or anuria for > 12 hrs

Loss:
Need of RRT for > 4 weeks

End-stage:
Need for RRT for > 3 months

Abbreviations: AKIN, Acute Kidney Injury Network; KDIGO, Kidney Disease: Improving Global Outcomes; RIFLE, risk, injury, failure, loss, and end-stage kidney disease; RRT, renal replacement therapy; SCr, serum creatinine.

[a]The urine output criteria for both the definition and staging of acute kidney injury are the same for the RIFLE, AKIN, and KDIGO criteria.

D. Cardiovascular disease.

E. Malignancy.

F. Liver disease.

G. Urological intervention.

(II) During a Hospital Admission

A. Surgery.

B. Sepsis.

C. Intravenous (IV) contrast.

D. > 20 mmHg decrease in blood pressure (BP).

E. Urinary obstruction.

F. Hypovolemia.

G. Malnourished.

(III) Nephrotoxins

A. Angiotensin converting enzyme inhibitors (ACEI)/angiotensin receptor blocker (ARBs).

B. Non-steroidal anti-inflammatory drugs, including cyclooxygenase 2 inhibitors.

C. Antivirals/antifungals.

D. Vancomycin/Gentamicin.

E. Chemotherapy/contrast medium.

(IV) Contrast Administration

If a patient is at risk (old, anemia, DM, congestive heart failure [CHF], CKD, hypotension, or repeat contrast use).

A. Mehran score for post-percutaneous coronary intervention contrast nephropathy risk [1].

B. Use iso- and low-osmolar contrast medium.
C. Minimize contrast volume.
D. IV 0.45% or 0.9% saline at the rate of 1 mL/kg/min from 12 hours before to 12 hours after the study.
E. No benefit of bicarbonate over IV saline [2].
F. No benefit of N-acetylcysteine [2].
G. Hold nonsteroidal anti-inflammatory drugs (NSAIDs).
H. No need to hold ACEI/ARBs [3].
I. No proven benefit of preemptive hemodialysis after contrast injection.

III. What Are Causes of AKI?

(I) Prerenal AKI

Renal hypoperfusion + preserved integrity of renal parenchyma tissue.

(II) Intrarenal (or intrinsic) AKI

Involving renal parenchymal tissue. Most intrinsic AKI is caused by ischemia or nephrotoxins, classically associated acute tubular necrosis (Table 11-2).

(III) Postrenal (or Obstructive) AKI

Acute obstruction of urinary tract.

(IV) Major Causes of Prerenal AKI

A. Intravascular Volume Depletion

(A) Hemorrhage: trauma, surgery, postpartum, gastrointestinal (GI).

(B) GI losses: diarrhea, vomiting, nasogastric drainage loss.

(C) Renal losses: diuretic use, osmotic diuresis, diabetes insipidus.

(D) Skin and mucous membrane losses: burns, hyperthermia.

(E) Nephrotic syndrome.

(F) Cirrhosis.

Table 11-2. Differential diagnosis of acute kidney injury

	Diagnostic index	Prerenal	ATN
Spot urine	FENa = (UNa/UCr)/(PNa/PCr) × 100%	< 1（鈉能回收）	> 1
	Urine sodium concentration (mmol/L)	< 10（鈉能回收）	> 20
	Urine to plasma urea nitrogen ratio	> 8	< 3
	Urine to plasma creatinine ratio	> 40	< 20
	Urine osmolality (mOsm/kgH$_2$O)	> 500（尿能濃縮）	~ 300
Serum	Plasma BUN/creatinine ratio	> 20	< 10–15
U/R	Urine specific gravity	> 1.020（尿能濃縮）	~1.010

[a]Acute glomerulonephritis, rhabdomyolysis, contrast-induced acute kidney injury may also present with a low FENa.

Abbreviations: ATN, acute tubular necrosis; BUN, blood urea nitrogen; FENa, fractional excretion of sodium.

B. Reduced Cardiac Output

(A) Cardiogenic shock.

(B) Pericardial diseases: restrictive, constricitve, tamponade.

(C) CHF.

(D) Valvular diseases.

(E) Pulmonary diseases: pulmonary hypertension, pulmonary embolism.

(F) Sepsis.

C. Systemic Vasodilation

(A) Sepsis

(B) Cirrhosis

(C) Anaphylaxis

(D) Drugs

D. Renal Vasocontriction

(A) Early sepsis.

(B) Hepatorenal syndrome.

(C) Acute hypercalcemia.

(D) Drugs: norepinephrine, vasopressin, NSAIDs, ACEI, calcineurin inhibitors.

(E) Iodinated contrast agents.

E. Increased Intraabdominal Pressure
(A) Abdominal compartment syndrome.

(V) Major Causes of Intrinsic AKI

A. Tubular Injury
(A) Ischemia and hypoperfusion: hypovolemia, sepsis, cirrhosis, CHF.
(B) Endogenous toxins: myoglobin, hemoglobin, paraproteinemia, uric acid.
(C) Exogenous toxins: chemotherapy, radiocontrast, phosphate preparations.

B. Tubulointerstitial Injury
(A) Acute allergic interstitial nephritis: NSAIDs, antibiotics (β-lactams), proton pump inhibitor.
(B) Infections: viral, bacterial, and fungal infections.
(C) Infiltration: lymphoma, leukemia, sarcoid.
(D) Allograft rejection.

C. Glomerular Injury
(A) Inflammation: anti-glomerular basement membrane, anti-neutrophil cytoplasmic antibody disease, infection, cryoglobulinemia, membranoproliferative glomerulonephritis, immunoglobulin A nephropathy, systemic lupus erythematosus, Henoch-Schonlein pupura, polyarteritis nodosa.
(B) Hemotologic: thrombotic microangiopathy, including hemolytic-uremic syndrome (HUS), atypical HUS, thrombotic thrombocytopenic purpura.

D. Renal Microvasculature
Malignant hypertension, preeclampsia, hypercalcemia, radiocontrast agents, scleroderma.

(VI) Major Causes of Post-renal AKI

A. Upper Urinary Tract Extrinsic Causes
(A) Retroperitoneal space: lymph nodes, tumors.
(B) Pelvic or intraabdominal tumors: cervix, uterus, ovary, prostate.
(C) Fibrosis: radiation, drugs, inflammation conditions.
(D) Ureteral ligation or surgical trauma.

(E) Granulomatosis diseases.

(F) Hematoma.

B. Upper Urinary Tract Intrinsic Causes

(A) Nephrolithiasis.

(B) Stricture.

(C) Edema.

(D) Debris, blood clots, sloughed papilla, fungal ball.

(E) Malignancy.

C. Lower Urinary Tract Causes

(A) Prostate: benign prostatic hyperplasia, carcinoma, infection.

(B) Bladder: neck obstruction, calculi, carcinoma, infection (schistosomiasis).

(C) Functional: neurogenic bladder, diabetes, multiple sclerosis, stoke, side effect of drugs (anticholinergics, antidepressants).

(D) Urethral: posterior urethral valves, strictures, trauma, tuberculosis, tumors.

IV. How to Assess/Monitor AKI?

(I) KDIGO Stage I

A. Obtain clinical history, check for risk factors, any pointers towards etiology, and review medications.

B. Clinical examination: fluid status (assess peripheral perfusion, jugular venous pressure, central venous pressure [CVP], edema, 3rd spacing accumulation), urine output.

C. Investigations: blood urea nitrogen (BUN)/Urea and electrolytes, urinalysis, chest X-Ray, electrocardiography (ECG).

D. Check arterial blood gas (ABG), lactate and anion gap (serum $[Na^+] + [K^+] - [Cl^-]$) if venous bicarbonate is low.

E. Consider renal ultrasound (US), sepsis screen.

(II) KDIGO Stage II

As for Stage I but renal US within 24 hours and sepsis screen.

(III) KDIGO Stage III

A. As for Stage II. Look for multi-organ failure and chase renal US report.
B. Mandatory blood tests: complete blood count, BUN/Urea, electrolytes, ABG, C-reactive protein, creatine kinase (rhabdomyolysis), liver function test (hepatorenal syndrome), prothrombin time and activated partial thromboplastin time.
C. Consider Lipase level, spot urine-to-creatinine ratio if proteinuria, autoantibody screen if hematuria or proteinuria, myeloma screen (Bence-Jones protein and serum free light chains), abdominal US.
(Note: AKI complications include: sepsis, acidosis, hyperkalemia, multi-organ failure, edema, respiratory failure, encephalopathy, hemorrhage.)

V. How to Treat AKI?

(I) Treat Underlying Disorder, Optimize Hemodynamics

(II) Correct Fluid Overload, Electrolyte and Acid-Base Imbalance

(III) Avoid Nephrotoxic Agents Use

(IV) Renal Support

A. KDIGO Stage I
(A) Avoid nephrotoxic agents exposure.
(B) Optimize fluid status.
(C) Correct hypovolemia, hydration, optimize hemodynamics, keep accurate fluid balance chart
   a. in severe sepsis, albumin in addition to crystalloids **did not** improve survival as compared with crystalloids alone [4].
   b. for critically ill intensive care unit (ICU) patients, risk of death and AKI was not lower with the use of balanced multielectrolyte solution than with saline [5].
(D) Treat infection if present.
(E) Relieve urinary obstruction if present.
(F) Fluid challenge unless there is evidence of fluid overload.
   Evaluation of fluid responsiveness: passive leg raising, pulse pressure variation, stroke volume variation, inferior vena cava diameter, end-expiratory occlusion test.

(G) Aim for mean BP > 65 or systolic blood pressure > 100 mmHg.

(H) Consider: vasoactive agents if hypotensive and not volume depleted.

(I) Assess response and follow up BUN/creatinine and electrolytes.

(J) Aim for urine output of 0.5 mL/kg/h.

(K) Consider: inserting urinary catheter, consider CVP for hemodynamic monitoring, review medication, and adjusting doses.

B. KDIGO Stage II

Manage as KDIGO Stage I and also:

(A) Insert urine catheter and check urine volumes hourly.

(B) Consider: CVP/cardiac monitoring, 12 hourly blood tests.

(C) Consult nephrologist if likely to need renal replacement therapy (RRT) or if no clinical improvement in 24–48 hours.

C. KDIGO Stage III

Manage as KDIGO Stage II and also:

(A) Consult nephrologist for possible RRT.

(B) Do cardiac monitoring.

(C) Consider: CVP line insertion and 12 hourly blood tests.

(D) Refer to ICU care if the patient is in respiratory failure or there is multi-organ involvement.

D. Referral Criteria to Nephrologist

(A) High suspicion of rapidly progressive glomerulonephritis.

(B) Indication for dialysis (refractory increase K^+ > 6.5 mmol/L, tumor lysis syndrome, refractory volume overload, refractory acidosis pH < 7.1, complications of uremia, severe poisoning, and severe hypothermia).

(C) Renal transplant patient.

VI. How to Manage AKI Complications?

(I) Hyperkalemia

A. ECG monitoring.

B. IV calcium gluconate 1–2 amp.
C. Insulin 10 U with 2–4 amp 50% dextrose IV drip over 15 minutes.
D. Salbutamol (Ventolin®) 10 mg nebulized (caution with salbutamol in tachycardia or ischemic heart disease).
E. If bicarbonate < 22 mmol/L and no fluid overload, consider IV sodium bicarbonate.
F. Diuretics and cation-exchanging resin (Kalimate®) use to lower total body potassium content.
G. Dialysis if intractable hyperkalemia.

(II) Metabolic Acidosis

A. Medical therapy of acidosis with bicarbonate should be reserved for emergency management of hyperkalemia.
B. ABG pH < 7.15 requires immediate critical care referral.
C. Dialysis if intractable acidosis.

(III) Pulmonary Edema

A. Oxygen supply, mechanical ventilation use if respiratory failure.
B. IV furosemide if hemodynamic stable. Consider repeat bolus and continuous infusion for better response.
C. Consider nitroglycerin 5 μg/min and titrating dose.
D. Dialysis if intractable fluid overloading.

(IV) Reduced Conscious Level (Uremic Encephalopathy)

A. Airway management
B. Critical care transfer
C. Urgent dialysis

(V) Hemorrhage (Uremic Bleeding)

A. Prolonged mechanical pressure over the bleeding area.
B. Consult specialists if endoscope is necessary (ear, nose and throat, GI, colon and rectal surgeons).
C. Management of anemia to keep Hb > 10 gm/dL.
D. Cryoprecipitate Infusion (8–12 U once).

E. Conjugated estrogen (Estromon® 5 tabs BID for 5 days).
F. Desmopressin:
   (A) Use in CKD patients with baseline serum creatinine > 4 mg/dL to avoid hyponatremia.
   (B) Desmopressin 4 amp in 50 mL N/S IV drip 30 mins.
G. Urgent dialysis if refractory to above therapy.

VII. What Are the Indications for Urgent Dialysis?

(I) Acid-base disorder: metabolic acidosis.
(II) Electrolyte disorder: hyperkalemia, hypercalcemia, tumor lysis.
(III) Intoxication: methanol, ethylene glycol, lithium, salicylates.
(IV) Overloading of fluid.
(V) Uremia: pericarditis, encephalopathy, bleeding.
   A. Above indications are conditions refractory to conventional therapy.
   B. Timing of initiation of RRT:
      (A) For critically ill sepsis patient with AKI, most evidence does not suggest mortality benefit for early (AKI diagnosed) vs. delayed initiation (presence of AEIOU) of RRT [6-8].
      (B) In severe AKI patients (oliguria > 72 hrs or BUN > 112 mg/dL), longer postponing of RRT initiation (more delayed vs. delayed strategy) did **not** confer additional benefit and was associated with potential harm [9].
      (C) For critically ill postoperative (especially open-heart surgery) patient with AKI, early initiation of RRT reduces mortality [10].

VIII. How to Differentiate Between AKI and CKD?

(I) History taking:
   Past CKD history, previous renal function tests, baseline creatinine.
(II) Lab exam:
   Anemia, high intact parathyroid hormone, radiological evidence of osteodystrophy (favor CKD).

(III) Renal sonography:

Chronic parenchymal change and small kidney size (normal kidney size:10–12 cm) (favor CKD).

CKD but with relative normal or large size of kidneys:

Diabetic nephropathy, human immunodeficiency virus nephropathy, polycystic kidney disease, amyloidosis, renal vein thrombosis, tumor infiltration.

參考文獻

[1] Mehran R, Aymong ED, Nikolsky E, et al. A simple risk score for prediction of contrast-induced nephropathy after percutaneous coronary intervention: development and initial validation. *J Am Coll Cardiol*. 2004;44(7):1393-1399. doi:10.1016/j.jacc.2004.06.068

[2] Weisbord SD, Gallagher M, Jneid H, et al. Outcomes after angiography with sodium bicarbonate and acetylcysteine. *N Engl J Med*. 2018;378(7):603-614. doi:10.1056/NEJMoa1710933

[3] Bainey KR, Rahim S, Etherington K, et al. Effects of withdrawing vs continuing renin-angiotensin blockers on incidence of acute kidney injury in patients with renal insufficiency undergoing cardiac catheterization: results from the Angiotensin Converting Enzyme Inhibitor/Angiotensin Receptor Blocker and Contrast Induced Nephropathy in Patients Receiving Cardiac Catheterization (CAPTAIN) trial. *Am Heart J*. 2015;170(1):110-116. doi:10.1016/j.ahj.2015.04.019

[4] Caironi P, Tognoni G, Masson S, et al. Albumin replacement in patients with severe sepsis or septic shock. *N Engl J Med*. 2014;370(15):1412-1421. doi:10.1056/NEJMoa1305727

[5] Finfer S, Micallef S, Hammond N, et al. Balanced multielectrolyte solution versus saline in critically ill adults. *N Engl J Med*. 2022;386(9):815-826. doi:10.1056/NEJMoa2114464

[6] STARRT-AKI Investigators; Canadian Critical Care Trials Group; Australian and New Zealand Intensive Care Society Clinical Trials Group; et al. Timing of initiation of renal-replacement therapy in acute kidney injury [published correction appears in *N Engl J Med*. 2020;383(5):502]. *N Engl J Med*. 2020;383(3):240-251. doi:10.1056/NEJMoa2000741

[7] Barbar SD, Clere-Jehl R, Bourredjem A, et al. Timing of renal-replacement therapy in patients with acute kidney injury and sepsis. *N Engl J Med*. 2018;379(15):1431-1442. doi:10.1056/NEJMoa1803213

[8] Gaudry S, Hajage D, Schortgen F, et al. Initiation strategies for renal-replacement therapy in the intensive care unit. *N Engl J Med*. 2016;375(2):122-133. doi:10.1056/NEJMoa1603017

[9] Gaudry S, Hajage D, Martin-Lefevre L, et al. Comparison of two delayed strategies for renal replacement therapy initiation for severe acute kidney injury (AKIKI 2): a multicentre, open-label, randomised, controlled trial. *Lancet*. 2021;397(10281):1293-1300. doi:10.1016/S0140-6736(21)00350-0

[10] Zarbock A, Kellum JA, Schmidt C, et al. Effect of early vs delayed initiation of renal replacement therapy on mortality in critically ill patients with acute kidney injury: the ELAIN randomized clinical trial. *JAMA*. 2016;315(20):2190-2199. doi:10.1001/jama.2016.5828

延伸閱讀資料

台灣腎臟醫學會。2020 台灣急性腎損傷處置共識。台灣急救加護醫學會。https://www.seccm.org.tw/files/index_iBook/iBook_001_2020%E6%80%A5%E6%80%A7%E8%85%8E%E6%90%8D%E5%82%B7%E8%99%95%E7%BD%AE.pdf

曾建華。Acute renal failure。於：曾建華。*First Choice 內專分科詳解*。臺北，臺灣：金名圖書；2011：158-160。

Ahn W, Radhakrishnan J, eds. *Pocket Nephrology*. 1st ed. Philadelphia, PA: Wolters Kluwer; 2020.

Gaudry S, Hajage D, Martin-Lefevre L, et al. Comparison of two delayed strategies for renal replacement therapy initiation for severe acute kidney injury (AKIKI 2): a multicentre, open-label, randomised, controlled trial. *Lancet*. 2021;397(10281):1293-1300. doi:10.1016/S0140-6736(21)00350-0

GGC Medicines-Adult Therapeutics Handbook. Management of Acute Kidney Injury (AKI). GGC Medicines-Adult Therapeutics Handbook Web site. https://handbook.ggcmedicines.org.uk/guidelines/renal/management-of-acute-kidney-injury-aki/. Updated March, 2023.

Jameson JL, Fauci AS, Kasper DL, Hauser SL, Longo DL, Loscalzo J, eds. *Harrison's Principles of Internal Medicine*. 20th ed. New York, NY: McGraw-Hill Education; 2018.

Yu ASL, Chertow GM, Luyckx V, Marsden PA, Skorecki K, Taal MW, eds. *Brenner and Rector's The Kidney*. 11th ed. Philadelphia, PA: Elsevier; 2019.

Chapter 12
Diabetic Kidney Disease

馬皓瑋
衛生福利部基隆醫院腎臟科
王植諄
三禾診所
黎思源
臺北榮民總醫院腎臟科

一、糖尿病的診斷與分類

(一) Criteria for the Diagnosis of Diabetes

符合下列至少一項，可考慮重複檢驗或使用二項以上確定診斷：
1. Glycated hemoglobin (HbA1c) ≥ 6.5%.
2. 空腹（至少 8 小時）血糖值 ≥ 126 mg/dL (7.0 mmol/L)。
3. 75 g 口服葡萄糖耐受測試後兩小時血糖值 ≥ 200 mg/dL (11.1 mmol/L)。
4. 出現典型高血糖症狀或發生高血糖急症合併隨機血糖值 ≥ 200 mg/dL。

(二) Classification

根據 2021 American Diabetes Association (ADA) guideline [1] 分類如下：
1. Type 1 diabetes.
2. Type 2 diabetes.
3. Specific types of diabetes due to other causes (e.g., monogenic diabetes syndromes, diseases of the exocrine pancreas, and drug/chemical-induced diabetes).
4. Gestational diabetes mellitus (DM).

二、糖尿病腎疾病 (Diabetic Kidney Disease, DKD) 的診斷

(一) 流行病學

慢性腎臟病 (chronic kidney disease, CKD) 藉由持續發生（大於三個月）的 albuminuria 與 glomerular filtration rate (GFR) 下降，或有其他腎臟損傷的證據診斷。DKD 指的是歸因於糖尿病的 CKD。約三分之一的糖尿病患者會發生糖尿病腎病變 (Type 1 DM: 25%–30%, Type 2 DM: 30%–40%)，這個比例在過去 20 年間並無太大變化，但由於全球糖尿病盛行率在這段期間不斷上升（尤其已開發國家），因此糖尿病腎病變的全球盛行率仍在上升，且為末期腎臟疾病 (end-stage kidney disease, ESKD) 的頭號原因。在糖尿病族群中，DKD 的發生，顯著增加心血管疾病的風險。

(二) 診斷及臨床進程

DKD 通常依靠臨床診斷。當糖尿病患者臨床上發現 albuminuria 及／或 GFR 的下降，符合 CKD 的診斷同時欠缺其它可能造成腎臟結構或功能受損的病因及表現，就會

考慮 DKD 的診斷。臨床線索包括長期的糖尿病、合併 diabetic retinopathy、缺少 gross hematuria 的 albuminuria 及漸進下降的 GFR。

典型的 DKD 臨床表現常在糖尿病診斷後約 10 年左右發現 albuminuria，且眼底鏡檢查出現糖尿病視網膜病變，後續合併 GFR 的下降（初期可能因 hyperfiltration 不減反增）；隨著時間進行，也可能伴隨水腫、高血壓甚至是腎病症候群等表現，並在糖尿病確診後 20 至 30 年間進展至 ESKD。在 Type 2 DM 患者身上，臨床進程常不呈現典型表現，包括糖尿病診斷當下已合併腎臟病變，也常發現診斷當下未合併視網膜病變或已發生 estimated glomerular filtration rate (eGFR) 下降卻無 albuminuria（Type 1 及 Type 2 DM 皆會發生，但 Type 2 DM 較常見）。

若臨床上發現腎功能或蛋白尿的快速惡化、出現 active urinary sediment、無法控制或快速惡化的高血壓、Type 1 DM 病患已發生腎功能異常卻缺少視網膜病變的證據或同時合併其他系統性疾病的臨床表現，需考慮其他可能的病因。在特定情況下 (Table 12-1)，需考慮進行腎臟切片協助鑑別診斷。

詳細的病史詢問與理學檢查是診斷 DKD 的基礎，病史詢問須包括詳細的發病過程、家族史、藥物史及有無其他系統性疾病病史。理學檢查則應注意糖尿病的小血管病變造成的變化，包括遠端脈搏減弱、皮膚傷口、潰瘍及任何神經學檢查發現。

若是新診斷的糖尿病且從年紀或臨床表現難以區分 Type 1 或 Type 2 DM，可考慮檢驗 C-peptide、glucagon stimulation test 協助鑑別 Type 1 與 Type 2 DM。若臨床上無法排除其它 primary/secondary glomerulonephritis，也須進行相關的檢驗，包括 C3/C4、immunoglobulins、anti-neutrophil cytoplasmic antibody、anti-GBM antibody、autoimmune disease markers、hepatitis B virus/hepatitis C virus/human immunodeficiency virus 等實驗室檢查。

（三）Albuminuria、GFR 與 Staging

檢驗隨機單次尿液 (random spot urine) 的 albumin 及 creatinine 相除以計算 urine albumin-to-creatinine ratio (UACR)，可有效代替 24 小時尿液檢查。依據 ADA 2021

Table 12-1. List of criteria for kidney biopsy in patients with diabetes

Criteria for kidney biopsy in patients with diabetes
1. Nephrotic range proteinuria or kidney failure in the absence of diabetic retinopathy
2. Nephrotic range proteinuria or kidney failure with diabetes duration less than 5 years
3. Nephrotic range proteinuria with normal kidney function
4. Unexplained microscopic hematuria or acute kidney injury
5. Rapidly worsening kidney function in patients with previously stable kidney function

guideline [1]，albuminuria 定義為 UACR ≥ 30 mg/g。傳統上可再區分為 microalbuminuria (30–300 mg/day) 及 macroalbuminuria (> 300 mg/g)。UACR 重複檢驗的變異性大，且容易受到發燒、感染、急性心臟衰竭、高血糖、嚴重高血壓、劇烈運動等因素影響，臨床上應考慮在 3 到 6 個月內重複檢驗 2 到 3 次以增加準確性。無論病患是否有糖尿病，白蛋白尿的發生皆是 cardiovascular (CV) mortality、all-cause mortality、cerebrovascular accident、GFR 下降及 ESKD 的強力預測因子。

GFR 通常藉由抽血檢驗 serum creatinine，並使用 Modification of Diet in Renal Disease (MDRD) 及 Chronic Kidney Disease Epidemiology Collaboration (CKD-EPI) 等公式計算 eGFR，一般認為 < 60 mL/min/1.73 m^2 為明顯異常。需要特別注意的是，在 DKD 早期常有 hyperfiltration 的現象，eGFR 往往不減反增，甚至可高達 180 mL/min/1.73 m^2，到病程晚期才出現快速的下降。

在臨床分期上，依照 The Kidney Disease: Improving Global Outcomes (KDIGO) 2012 CKD guideline [2] 的 CKD 預後分級，以 GFR (G1–G5) 及 albuminuria (A1–A3) 的程度區分。這樣的分級主要提供的是預後指標，包括急性腎損傷、all-cause mortality、CV mortality、CKD progression 及 ESKD 的風險程度，但無法直接對應不同的臨床治療策略。

（四）Risk Factors

糖尿病患者發生 DKD 的可能危險因子如 Table 12-2 所示。其中有些危險因子較為顯著，如糖尿病診斷時間、高血糖與高血壓廣泛被認為對於 DKD 的發生與進展有極大影響；有些危險因子則較不明確或僅限於特定族群，如蛋白質攝取及某些特定基因。臨床上須針對可改變之危險因子以藥物或生活方式進行介入，以減少 DKD 的發生或進展。

Table 12-2. Risk factors of diabetic kidney disease

Duration of DM	Insulin resistance
Hyperglycemia	Pregnancy
Hypertension	Intrauterine factors
Hyperfiltration	Smoking
Dyslipidemia	Periodontal disease
Dietary protein	Cardiac autonomic neuropathy
Obesity	Genetic factors

Abbreviation: DM, diabetes mellitus.

（五）Pathology

DKD 表現的腎臟病理變化相當多變，且臨床上常合併其他腎絲球病變的病理變化。典型的 DKD 腎絲球病灶如 Table 12-3 所示，除了協助隨著分級的進行可能反映隨著時間進行的疾病進程，配合 interstitial 及 vascular 的病理變化也可能對 CKD progression 等 outcome 有預測價值。Type 1 DM 較常出現典型的病理變化及進程，而 Type 2 DM 的病理表現則較常有極大的變異性，包括可能與腎絲球變化比例不符的間質或血管病灶；這樣的差異可能與 Type 2 DM 病患常合併其他病因有關，如高血壓、老化、肥胖。

三、Management

DKD 的治療主要可分成生活型態的介入，以及針對高血糖、高血壓、蛋白尿以及血脂異常等 DKD 危險因子的藥物治療兩大類。KDIGO 2020 [3] 強調同時考慮減緩 CKD progression 風險及心血管風險的 comprehensive strategy (Figure 12-1)。

（一）Protein and Sodium Intake

針對蛋白質攝取，建議非透析的 CKD 病患維持約每日每 kg 體重 0.8 g 的蛋白質攝取量。高蛋白飲食（大於每日每 kg 體重 1.3 g）與腎功能與蛋白尿的惡化直接相關，也

Table 12-3. Classification of diabetic kidney disease glomerular lesions

Class	Description	Inclusion Criteria
I	Mild or nonspecific LM changes and EM-proven GBM thickening	• Biopsy does not meet class II, III, or IV • GBM > 395 nm in female • GBM > 430 nm in male
IIa	Mild mesangial expansion	• Biopsy does not meet class III or IV • Mild mesangial expansion in > 25% of the observed mesangium
IIb	Severe mesangial expansion	Severe mesangial expansion in > 25% of the observed mesangium
III	Nodular sclerosis (K-W lesion)	• Biopsy does not meet criteria for class IV • At least one convincing K-W lesion
IV	Advanced diabetic glomerulosclerosis	Global glomerular sclerosis in > 50% of glomeruli

Abbreviations: EM, electron microscopy; GBM, glomerular basement membrane ; K-W lesion, Kimmelstiel-Wilson lesion; LM, light microscopy.

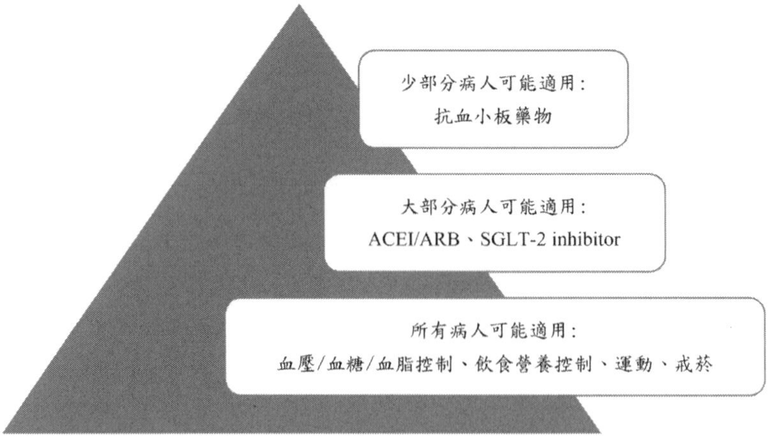

```
                少部分病人可能適用:
                   抗血小板藥物

            大部分病人可能適用:
            ACEI/ARB、SGLT-2 inhibitor

        所有病人可能適用:
        血壓/血糖/血脂控制、飲食營養控制、運動、戒菸
```

Figure 12-1. Kidney–heart risk factor management

Abbreviations: ACEI, angiotensin converting enzyme inhibitors; ARB, angiotensin receptor blocker; SGLT-2, sodium-glucose cotransporter 2.

有較差的心血管預後,需要避免。而小於每日每 kg 體重 0.8 g 的蛋白質攝取量的效益則缺乏實證,且有可能造成營養不良,因此不被建議。鹽份的攝取則建議控制在每日小於 2,300 mg 的鈉攝取量,相當於 6 g 以下食鹽,對血壓的控制及心血管預後有幫助。

(二) Glycemic Control

隨著腎功能的下降,尤其 eGFR < 60 mL/min/1.73 m² 後,會造成胰島素及口服血糖藥的代謝能力下降,再加上腎臟本身為 gluconeogenesis 的重要器官(約占全身 40%),發生低血糖的風險會逐漸升高,因此在處方降血糖藥物時須特別注意藥物的作用時間、代謝途徑、禁忌症及副作用,避免低血糖的發生。無論採用何種降血糖藥物治療,臨床醫師須至少每三到六個月重新評估藥物的使用及劑量。以下簡單介紹目前各種降血糖藥物在糖尿病腎病變病患身上的應用。

1. Human insulin and analogs:又可分為速效(如:aspart、lispro)、短效(如 human regular)、中長效(如 neutral protamine Hagedorn [NPH])及長效(如 detemir、glargine、degludec)。處方時須注意 CKD 病患胰島素的代謝能力下降會造成藥物作用的時間延長,如劑量或頻次不適當可能會造成低血糖。Human insulin(如 NPH)可能比 insulin analog 有更高的低血糖風險。胰島素除了對血糖的控制,無額外的 CV/renal benefits。幾乎所有 Type 1 DM 患者在診斷時就須接受胰島素治療。

2. Sulfonylurea (SU):第一代 SU 現在幾乎已不再使用,現存的 SU 為第二代(如 glipizide、glimepiride),作用時間較短,發生低血糖的風險較低,但在晚期 CKD

及透析病患身上依然存有代謝時間延長的問題，因此現今較少使用在晚期 CKD 或透析病患身上。

3. Meglitinide：作用機轉與 SU 相似，但作用時間比 SU 更短。其中 repaglinide 主要經肝臟代謝，在 CKD 晚期或透析病患身上使用安全性更高，與降血脂藥物 gemfibrozil 併用時藥物濃度會升高造成低血糖風險上升，需注意避免併用。

4. Biguanide：目前僅 metformin 在市面上販售，在大部分情況下仍為 Type 2 DM 的第一線口服降血糖藥。Metformin 主要經腎臟排除，使用在 advanced CKD 病患身上會大幅提高發生 lactate acidosis 的風險，KDIGO 2020 guideline 建議 eGFR < 45 mL/min/1.73 m^2 須減半劑量，< 30 mL/min/1.73 m^2 或透析病患則應停藥，U.S. Food and Drug Administration 也將 eGFR < 30 mL/min/1.73 m^2 列為禁忌症。Metformin 對於 atherosclerotic cardiovascular disease (ASCVD) 可能有潛在好處。

5. Thiazolidinedione：主要經由肝臟代謝，但有可能會增加腎小管對鈉和水的再吸收，而造成水腫與心衰竭，同時也有可能造成 bone formation 減少與 bone loss 增加而提高骨折的發生率，一般來說不建議用在糖尿病腎病變病患身上。

6. α-glucosidase inhibitor：雖然此類藥物僅微量會被腸胃道吸收，但血中濃度在 CKD 病患身上會升高，一般不建議 eGFR < 30 mL/min/1.73 m^2 之病患使用。

7. Dipeptidyl peptidase 4 (DPP4) inhibitor：藉由抑制 DPP-IV 作用延長 glucagon-like peptide-1 (GLP-1) 作用時間而刺激胰島素分泌並抑制 glucagon 分泌。與 SU 相比，此類藥物對於 β cell 的刺激作用需依賴血中葡萄糖，因此血糖較低時效果會減弱，減少了低血糖的風險。Sitagliptin 與 saxagliptin 須依據 eGFR 調整劑量，linagliptin 則不需調整劑量。此類藥物無獨立於血糖控制外的 CV/renal benefits，saxagliptin 可能會增加心臟衰竭的風險。由於機轉重疊，不建議與 GLP-1 receptor agonist (GLP-1 RA) 合併使用。

8. GLP-1 RA：臺灣現有 exenatide、liraglutide、dulaglutide、semaglutide、lixisenatide 等針劑可使用。Lixisenatide 及 exenatide 目前不建議用於 eGFR < 30 mL/min/1.73 m^2 之患者。Liraglutide、dulaglutide、semaglutide 有對於 ASCVD 的額外好處，也可能減緩 DKD 的進展。GLP-1 RA 也有一定的減重效果，且對於血糖控制的效果佳，因此對於口服降血糖藥無法達到 HbA1c 控制目標而需要針劑治療的病患，ADA 2021 guideline 建議可考慮 GLP-1 RA 優先於 basal insulin，也可考慮併用 basal insulin 治療。使用上須特別考慮腸胃道副作用（雖然可能帶來體重減輕的好處），並逐步增加治療劑量。

9. Sodium-glucose cotransporter-2 (SGLT2) inhibitor：藉由抑制主要分布於近曲小管 (proximal convoluted tubule) 前段上皮細胞的 SGLT2，SGLT2 inhibitor 可直接造成每

Chapter 12 Diabetic Kidney Disease

日 40–80 g 的葡萄糖經由尿液排出體外,並減輕體重,其作用並不直接影響胰島素生成與代謝,因此不會造成低血糖,且可與其他口服血糖藥併用。此類藥物臺灣現有 empagliflozin、dapagliflozin、canagliflozin,皆已被大型 randomized controlled trial 證實能有效減少 Type 2 DM 病患心臟衰竭及 CKD 惡化之風險。除了藉由血糖控制與減輕體重減緩胰島素阻抗性並改善 β-cell 功能外,此類藥物還有眾多可能幫助改善心臟及腎臟預後的機轉。輕微的滲透性利尿及直接的利鈉效果,可能協助改善血壓;藉由減少鈉的再吸收及調控 tubuloglomerular feedback,減緩腎絲球 hyperfiltration 並改善腎臟組織缺氧;藉由刺激腎臟局部 hypoxia-inducible factors 的產生改善腎性貧血。以上機轉可能直接或間接改善心血管及腎臟預後,且部分益處可能不會隨著 GFR 的下降減弱。根據 ADA 2022 guideline,Type 2 DM 病患除生活型態改善及 metformin 治療,若合併 heart failure、CKD、ASCVD 或有相關疾病的高風險且須使用第二種降血糖藥物治療,應優先考慮 SGLT2 inhibitor(合併 ASCVD 也可考慮 GLP-1 RA)。使用此類藥物皆須注意依據腎功能調整劑量,並視不同藥物在特定 eGFR 以下停藥,也得注意 diabetic ketoacidosis 或泌尿道感染等風險。

DKD 的血糖控制流程建議如 Figure 12-2。

(三) Glycemic Target

早期糖尿病治療指引一般建議 intensive glycemic control (HbA1c = 7%),可能減少糖尿病的小血管病變,但較嚴格的血糖控制也帶來較高的低血糖風險。KDIGO 2020 [3] 不指定單一特定血糖控制目標,強調應針對不同病患設定個人化 HbA1c target (6.5%–8%)。常見須考量因素如 Table 12-4 所示。

(四) 血壓控制與 Renin-Angiotensin System (RAS) Blockade

依據現行治療指引及大型研究,對於所有未合併發生 albuminuria 的糖尿病及 DKD 病患,血壓應至少控制在 < 140/90 mmHg;若合併 albuminuria,進一步控制在 < 130/80 mmHg 可能有額外好處。Angiotensin converting enzyme inhibitors (ACEI) 或 angiotensin receptor blocker (ARB) 應該作為第一線治療用藥,以減低心血管風險並減緩蛋白尿惡化;若無法達標,可考慮加上 calcium-channel blockers 及利尿劑等藥物。針對血壓正常但合併 albuminuria 的糖尿病患者,也應考慮使用 ACEI/ARB 治療。短暫的 serum creatinine 上升可能出現在新使用 ACEI/ARB 或增加劑量的患者,如四週內 creatinine 未上升超過 30%,可繼續使用。針對腎功能較差的患者,須特別注意可能發生高血鉀。針對沒有高血壓也無 albuminuria 的糖尿病患者,目前不建議使用 RAS blockade 作為 DKD primary prevention。

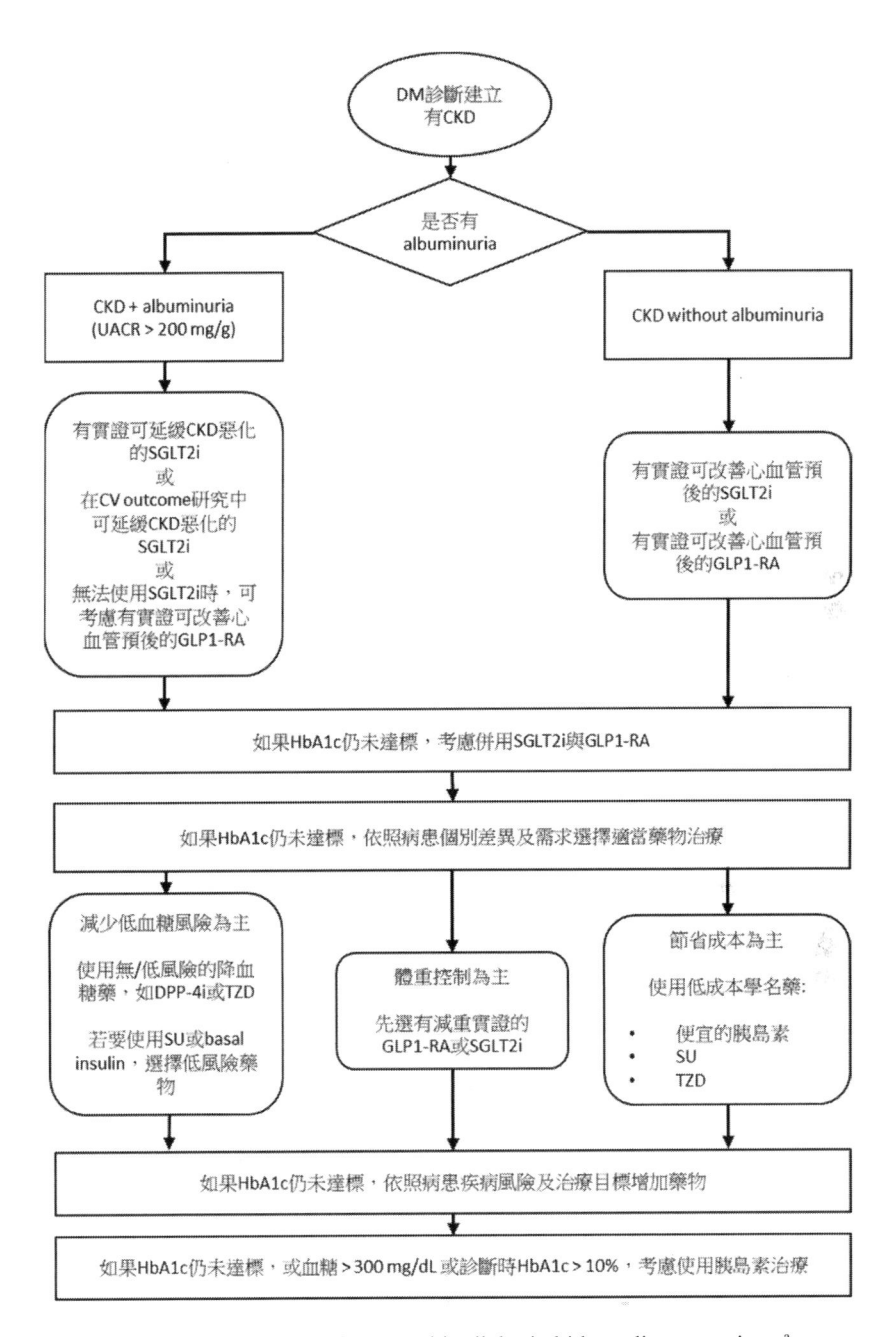

Figure 12-2. Glycemic control in diabetic kidney disease patients[a]

Abbreviations: UACR, urine albumin-to-creatinine ratio; HbA1c, glycated hemoglobin; CKD, chronic kidney disease; CV, cardiovascular; DM, diabetes mellitus; DPP-4i, dipeptidyl peptidase 4 inhibitor; GLP1-RA, GLP-1 receptor agonist; SGLT2i, sodium-glucose cotransporter-2 inhibitor; SU, sulfonylurea; TZD, thiazolidinedione.

[a] 資料參考來源：[4]。

Chapter 12 Diabetic Kidney Disease

Table 12-4. 個人化 HbA1c 目標的主要決定因素

個人化 HbA1c 目標	較嚴格 (6.5%) ←——→ 較寬鬆 (8.0%)	
CKD 嚴重度	低	高
大血管併發症	少／輕微	多／嚴重
共病症	少	多
預期壽命	長	短
低血糖自我警覺能力	完整	喪失
低血糖醫療照護可近性	好	差
個人低血糖發生傾向	少	多

Abbreviations: HbA1c, glycated hemoglobin; CKD, chronic kidney disease.

（五）Lipid-Lowering Therapy

所有 40–75 歲 DM 患者皆應使用 moderate-intensity statin 藥物作為初級預防，減少 ASCVD 風險及相關死亡；如合併兩項以上 ASCVD 風險因子（DM > 10 years，UACR > 30 mg/g、eGFR < 60 mL/min/1.73 m^2，眼底或神經病變，ankle-brachial index < 0.9）則須使用 high-intensity statin 治療。如病患合併難以控制之 hypertriglyceridemia 也可考慮加上 fenofibrate 或 niacin 等藥物。合併使用 statin 與 fibrate 會增加 rhabdomyolysis 的發生率，如病患需合併用藥需小心監測副作用。

四、Special Consideration

（一）Metabolic Acidosis

糖尿病腎病變是造成 Type IV renal tubular acidosis 最常見的原因，必要時須使用口服 sodium bicarbonate 控制 HCO$_3^-$ level，避免酸血症進一步惡化腎功能。若合併高血鉀則需使用降鉀藥物控制，並謹慎 ACEI/ARB 等可能造成高血鉀的藥物。

（二）Acute Kidney Injury

糖尿病腎病變患者較容易因 iodinated contrast exposure、non-steroidal anti-inflammatory drug 或 volume depletion 而發生急性腎損傷，需特別注意。臨床上改善可能造成 DKD 的危險因子也可能同時減少發生急性腎損傷之風險。

（三）Dialysis

1. Hemodialysis：糖尿病患者容易合併大血管病變，周邊血管狀況往往較其他腎臟病患者為差，如病患考慮接受血液透析，要儘早評估是否能建立適當的血管通路。
2. Peritoneal dialysis：含葡萄糖之透析液會對糖尿病患之血糖、血脂控制與體重產生不良影響，如病患考慮接受腹膜透析，治療過程要特別注意血糖及血脂藥物的調整。此副作用相較於血液透析是否會對病患存活率有負面影響目前仍有爭議。若使用icodextrin成分之腹膜透析液，須特別注意可能對特定血糖檢驗方式產生誤差。

參考文獻

[1] American Diabetes Association. 2. Classification and diagnosis of diabetes: standards of medical care in diabetes—2021 [published correction appears in *Diabetes Care*. 2021;44(9):2182]. *Diabetes Care*. 2021;44(Suppl 1):S15-S33. doi:10.2337/dc21-S002

[2] Kidney Disease: Improving Global Outcomes (KDIGO) CKD Work Group. KDIGO 2012 clinical practice guideline for the evaluation and management of chronic kidney disease. *Kidney Int Suppl*. 2013;3(1):1-150.

[3] Kidney Disease: Improving Global Outcomes (KDIGO) Diabetes Work Group. KDIGO 2020 clinical practice guideline for diabetes management in chronic kidney disease. *Kidney Int*. 2020;98(4S):S1-S115. doi:10.1016/j.kint.2020.06.019

[4] American Diabetes Association Professional Practice Committee. 11. Chronic kidney disease and risk management: standards of medical care in diabetes–2022 [published correction appears in *Diabetes Care*. 2022;45(3):758] [published correction appears in *Diabetes Care*. 2022;45(9):2182-2184]. *Diabetes Care*. 2022;45(Suppl 1):S175-S184. doi:10.2337/dc22-S011

延伸閱讀文獻

Taal MW. Chapter 59. Classification and Management of Chronic Kidney Disease In: Taal MW, Chertow GM, Marsden PA, Skorecki K, Yu ASL, Brenner BM, eds. *Brenner and Rector's the Kidney*. 9th ed. Philadelphia, PA: Elsevier; 2011:1659-1675

American Diabetes Association. Standards of medical care in diabetes—2022. *Diabetes Care*. 2022;45(Suppl 1):S1-S264.

Fornoni A, Nelson RG, Najafian B, Groop PH. Epidemiology of diabetic kidney disease. In: Yu ASL, Chertow GM, Luyckx VA, Marsden PA, Skorecki K, Taal MW, eds. *Brenner & Rector's. The Kidney*. 11th ed. Philadelphia, PA: Elsevier; 2020:1327-1379

Kidney Disease: Improving Global Outcomes (KDIGO) Blood Pressure Work Group. KDIGO clinical practice guideline for the management of blood pressure in chronic kidney disease. *Kidney Int Suppl*. 2012;2(5):337-414.

Kidney Disease: Improving Global Outcomes (KDIGO) Diabetes Work Group. KDIGO 2020 clinical practice guideline for diabetes management in chronic kidney disease. *Kidney Int*. 2020;98(4S):S1-S115. doi:10.1016/j.kint.2020.06.019

Kitabchi AE, Umpierrez GE, Miles JM, Fisher JN. Hyperglycemic crises in adult patients with diabetes. *Diabetes Care*. 2009;32(7):1335-1343. doi:10.2337/dc09-9032

Rhee CM, Leung AM, Kovesdy CP, Lynch KE, Brent GA, Kalantar-Zadeh K. Updates on the management of diabetes in dialysis patients. *Semin Dial*. 2014;27(2):135-145. doi:10.1111/sdi.12198

Tuttle KR, Bakris GL, Bilous RW, et al. Diabetic kidney disease: a report from an ADA Consensus Conference. *Diabetes Care*. 2014;37(10):2864-2883. doi:10.2337/dc14-1296

國家圖書館出版品預行編目（CIP）資料

腎臟醫學臨床技能手冊 = The handbook of clinical skills in nephrology / 牛志遠, 王宗悅, 王植諄, 何揚, 吳采虹, 李宗翰, 李國華, 李景伯, 沈書慧, 周以新, 林志慶, 林堯彬, 胡譯安, 唐德成, 馬皓瑋, 莊喬琳, 陳紀瑜, 陳進陽, 陳範宇, 曾偉誠, 楊晴涵, 楊智宇, 歐朔銘, 蔡友蓮, 蔡明村, 黎思源作；唐德成, 林志慶主編. -- 第二版. -- 華藝數位股份有限公司學術出版部出版：華藝數位股份有限公司發行, 2023.06

面： 公分
ISBN 978-986-437-206-5(平裝)
1.CST: 腎臟疾病 2.CST: 臨床醫學
415.84　　　　　　　　　　　　　　112007687

腎臟醫學臨床技能手冊 第二版
The Handbook of Clinical Skills in Nephrology, 2nd Edition

主　　編／唐德成、林志慶
副 主 編／曾偉誠、簡志潁
作　　者／牛志遠、王宗悅、王植諄、何揚、吳采虹、李宗翰、李國華、李景伯、沈書慧、
　　　　　周以新、林志慶、林堯彬、胡譯安、唐德成、馬皓瑋、莊喬琳、陳紀瑜、陳進陽、
　　　　　陳範宇、曾偉誠、楊晴涵、楊智宇、歐朔銘、蔡友蓮、蔡明村、黎思源
　　　　　（依姓氏筆劃排序）

責任編輯／張育閑
封面設計／張大業
版面編排／王凱倫

發 行 人／常效宇
總 編 輯／張慧銖
業　　務／陳姍儀
出　　版／華藝數位股份有限公司　學術出版部（Ainosco Press）
　　　　　地址：234 新北市永和區成功路一段 80 號 18 樓
　　　　　電話：(02)2926-6006　傳真：(02)2923-5151
　　　　　服務信箱：press@airiti.com
發　　行／華藝數位股份有限公司
　　　　　戶名（郵局／銀行）：華藝數位股份有限公司
　　　　　郵政劃撥帳號：50027465
　　　　　銀行匯款帳號：0174440019696（玉山商業銀行　埔墘分行）
法律顧問／立暘法律事務所　歐宇倫律師
Ｉ Ｓ Ｂ Ｎ／978-986-437-206-5
Ｄ　Ｏ　Ｉ／10.978.986437/2065
出版日期／2023 年 6 月（第二版）
定　　價／新台幣 480 元

版權所有・翻印必究
（如有缺頁或破損，請寄回本社更換，謝謝）